Justice in Health

Camille Burnett

Justice in Health

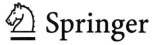 Springer

Camille Burnett
Burnett Innovation LLC
Richmond, VA, USA

ISBN 978-3-031-18506-9   ISBN 978-3-031-18504-5   (eBook)
https://doi.org/10.1007/978-3-031-18504-5

This Springer imprint is published by the registered company Springer Nature Switzerland AG
The registered company address is: Gewerbestrasse 11, 6330 Cham, Switzerland

Preface

The greatest opportunity we have to transform health is to democratize and liberate it through unencumbered imagination, innovation, and, quite frankly, courage. Most telling of the need to do this is recognizing that what we are doing is not working. Yet, we are continuing to do it. Evidence of the lack of success in our health "doing" is increasing health disparities and widening life expectancy gaps and critical system failures in capacity and access. We see overt and covert acts of racism (personal, institutional, structural, and cultural); experience escalating violence in mass shooting, interpersonally and within neighborhoods; and increasing infringement on the most basic of human rights (voting, abortion, and dignity). The health of the nation and our communities is at stake. The health of our patients and clients being served is at stake. The healthcare profession's credibility and functionality are at stake. We are literally in a crisis of health, health integrity, and health consciousness in this country. We are facing an existential threat to our humanity.

The alarm has been sounded in various ways, and we cannot continue to ignore it by "back-burnering" these intersectional issues we face. The pandemics (COVID-19, racism, and social unrest) we have experienced and continue to experience have spoken loudly. They have told us that there are consequences to inaction and that there is an interconnectedness of issues and of each other. The consequences of failing to address racism and health disparities exacerbated the prevalence, morbidity, and mortality of COVID-19, impacting the health system, the economy, and our mental health. There will never be an "after COVID" moment. We crossed an invisible precipice at the height of the pandemics that we cannot undo, ever. The entire world was simultaneously for the most part under some form of quarantine that allowed everyone to take a collective pause. During the pause, people's attention was captured in ways that the *business as usual* lifestyle we were living up to that point did not allow. It opened up space to reflect on life, for self-examination and for re-invention.

In the United States, this pause also fell during the publicized successive killing of Black people, and in particular, we watched the murdering of George Floyd, Breonna Taylor, Ahmaud Arbery and many others. While unjust killing of Black and Brown bodies has been going on for generations, the actual moments being visually captured and televised rocked our collective souls. For some, unseeing what was seen has not been possible and this too was the case for the healthcare profession who also witnessed the disproportionate COVID-19 deaths among First Nations, Latinx, and Black populations. All of this has been too much. At the same time, the scourge of racism, health disparities, and inequities are not new. They have been known. That is the greatest travesty of it all. The decades of inaction and complacency of our systems, institutions, and policies are appalling. Shaming and blaming at this point is not helpful. People have died and are continuing to die even as this book is being written. Expeditious solutions and actions are what is needed, which is what this book hopes to provide. Contextualized knowledge with action to rectify and transform health care in the United States by providing more than a textbook of health equity information is what this book is about. Textbooks, although informative, can feel antiquated and removed from the current reality. *Justice in Health* is a guide, a road map, and a strategic manual offering bold thought leadership in delicate but necessary aspects and narratives of health. There is some historically significant information provided throughout that serves to situate and explain that which might seem random. Nothing is random, and the root cause of all health inequities should be illuminated to build the platform to reform, restore, and rectify. It is where justice in health begins.

Delving into root causes forces us to reflect on history and narratives that are foundational to our epistemological and ontological understanding of our profession and how to move forward in the world we are experiencing now. To get there, *Justice in Health* starts the conversation in Chap. 1 with unpacking the most basic, overused, and arguably least consistently understood term—health. In general, healthcare providers have simply accepted the idea of a shared understanding of health either within their discipline or across their discipline. Furthermore, health disciplines were formed based on previous definitions of what health is while practicing within very different parameters now. While the meaning of health has changed, health discipline practices and systems have lagged. Similarly, those outside of the health arena have also assumed a shared understanding of health that has been translated into mandates, policies, and systems. Knowing this is important because if there is not a collective understanding of health, a disconnect is created between what we think health is and how it is experienced, which misleads our solutions. *Justice in Health* attempts to unpack the definition of health, to realign it to create not only consistency in our understanding of what health is contextualized within the present but also to inform equitable and just solutions that work. Workable, equitable, and just solutions are those that speak to structures at the intersection of health and humanity and seek to answer questions that this book attempts to answer such as what it will take from an imagination, innovation, and courageous perspective to attain justice in health.

Each chapter of this book provides insights toward the achievement of justice in health, posing thought-provoking considerations of what it could be. Chapter 1 provides an overview and global introduction to the book's content. In the introduction, understanding of core concepts of public health, equity, justice, and health are established. This chapter centers on unpacking the meaning of health, how health is understood and misunderstood, and, most importantly, how health is created. Its impact in producing outcomes across the determinants of health is examined across an ecological spectrum of the populations, communities, and the system of care. The conceptual exploration of just health and what the creation of a more just system of health means will be introduced and situated in relation to our society and why health matters.

Chapter 2 helps to contextualize and situate race and health in the United States. It recognizes that in the United States and even globally, we face ever-increasing health disparities and widening inequality gaps especially among Black, Brown, Asian, Latinx, and Indigenous peoples. These populations have historically and intentionally been subjugated, excluded, and marginalized, causing generational devastation to their social, economic, and health outcomes. Routinely, racialized populations disproportionately suffer from higher rates of negative health-related sequela (health disparities, chronic disease, morbidity, and mortality) and disparate social consequences (such as poverty, limited access to opportunity, decrease social mobility, and racism) that diminish life expectancy and quality of life. Direct and indirect impacts of cumulative and intersecting exposure to these consequences produce chronic challenges that are further exacerbated by structures (institutions, policies, practices, and institutional agents), and the inequitable distribution of power and privilege and the history of race and health in this country are examined.

Chapter 3 delves into frameworks for situating justice in health with a deeply philosophical introduction and exploration of key theories most critical to meet the health and well-being challenges we face as a nation in this moment. Highlighted are discussions of critical theories and perspectives that include but are not limited to postcolonial and emancipatory inquiry, social justice in nursing practice, structural violence, and structural justice. Discussions about the social determinants of health are at the forefront to help introduce the reader to contextual causes that determine health guided by these various theoretical perspectives. This chapter serves to synthesize structural and root causes through a theoretical landscape to expose the hidden realities of power, privilege, and social identity.

In Chap. 4, we dive into health equity and critical health issues by unpacking critical root causes that perpetuate health disparities such as race, poverty, mass and youth incarceration, and violence against women, communities, and society. It also examines issues that determine health such as access to care, food, housing, transportation, and insurance using concrete examples. Beyond identification of these issues, this chapter makes the connection to earlier perspectives discussed in Chap. 3 to extend and situate health in relation to structural drivers and root causes. It is connecting the dots beyond the current healthcare orientation that leads to a deepening of understanding of how health happens across disparate populations and in aggregate populations. It also begins to frame what a health equity systems approach could look like and what must be considered.

Chapter 5 starts to explore how to create a healthcare system without walls to build a culture of healing. This chapter reframes the current beliefs of what a healthcare system is, toward what it could be within the concept of building a system of care without walls. A healthcare system without walls is discussed by identifying structural obstacles and gaps within the current structure including their impacts and introducing new ways to overcome and dismantle these challenges. A core pillar in this discussion is critical conversations about what it means to be a healthcare provider and how we can better prepare healthcare providers to meet the demands of a new re-imagined system. To this end, the chapter also introduces trauma-informed and healing approaches, one of the key professional shifts required in the routine preparation of healthcare providers. As an overarching mechanism for facilitating healing, this chapter covers understanding trauma, its consequences, and its impacts at an individual and community level. It examines what a culture of healing looks like through a trauma-informed orientation and explores the healing of individuals and communities who have experienced trauma. The core elements of a trauma-informed approach and their application across this spectrum, which will include recommendations and useful approaches to implementing a culture of healing, are provided.

Chapter 6 advocates leading through just action by introducing readers to community engagement and partnerships as facilitators to rebuilding and co-creating a renewed system of care. Understanding community partnerships and their importance is discussed. Examining practice partnerships and best practice approaches for engaging with the community to meet their health needs where they are is a central component of this chapter. The chapter draws on community engagement and partnership examples from the field that have been used to demonstrate how communities can mobilize and transform health. It also discusses the use and power of platforms such as media for advocacy and use of data as tools for change. The chapter will serve to help health providers, health researchers, and health educators consider non-traditional approaches to creatively find ways to exchange knowledge, skills, and expertise needed to reform and redress health disparities. It is a chapter that encourages healthcare providers to act effectively to create and influence equitable health solutions.

The book concludes with Chap. 7, "Just Health," that serves to summarize and synthesize the important points, complexitie,s and concepts raised throughout the previous chapters. It culminates in a discussion that pays particular attention to upstream versus downstream public and population health approaches to make the case as to why the reconciliation of public health toward just health cannot wait. Just health is revisited against this backdrop and summarized at the praxis of theory, knowledge, and action toward achieving health justice. The chapter concludes with a call to action and suggested steps to address the urgent and emergent conditions that mitigate health outcomes and identify opportunities for change that can be leveraged now. It can be used to fuel galvanized action that serves as the impetus for a new health justice movement in this country.

Revisiting the earlier assertion of this book, its charge is to examine and interrogate the intersection of health and humanity with the anticipation of not only inspiring minds but also to prepare healthcare providers with fundamental knowledge to transform their practice. It is hoped that students, faculty, and administrators will reflect on the question of what it will take for us to imagine and innovate something different and do we have the courage to try. If all of us ask this question, this book will serve to guide you through options and approaches to help you formulate your own action plan with a collective aim to achieve justice in health.

Richmond, VA, USA   Camille Burnett

Acknowledgments

With gratitude I thank the creative being who inspired my calling and gifted me with innovative thinking, an astute ability to envision, and humility to learn and embrace all forms of knowledge for the betterment of humanity.

I am grateful to my beautiful family and circle of colleagues affectionately known as my tribe both near and far who inspire and amaze me every day.

Thank you to the Springer family for encouraging me and enthusiastically supporting what has been a truly remarkable endeavor, and to my research support personnel for your contributions in summarizing parts of the US and global healthcare systems' discussion and history of nursing theory information.

Contents

About the Author

Camille Burnett, **PhD**, **MPA**, **APHN-BC**, **RN**, **BSc.N**, **DSW**, **CGNC**, **FAAN**, is a *social innovator and thought leader* whose work critically addresses the social and structural drivers of health, equity, and structural justice. Dr. Burnett is the founder and principal of Burnett Innovation LLC, and provides expertise in public health, health equity, health policy, and health and structural justice. Dr. Burnett educates, conducts research and evaluation and oversees health equity and population health initiative. She aligns these efforts toward the co-creation of health equity and innovative justice solutions that attend to structural and policy drivers of health and opportunity for overlooked and excluded populations.

Dr. Burnett has extensive professional experience within the US and Canadian healthcare systems; in academia, public health, public health management, and research; and as a private consultant. She has held provincial public health administrator leadership positions in Canada and academic administrator leadership positions in the United States. Dr. Burnett has held community engagement and service appointments on a multitude of local, national, and international boards, and selected appointments as a national policy think tank appointee and internationally as one of only 30 International Council of Nursing 2019 Global Nurse Leaders. Dr. Burnett holds several professional affiliations; is the recipient of 21 teaching excellence awards and four university-wide teaching awards; has published more than 22 scientific articles, 4 book chapters, 1 book and has been highlighted in several media stories; and participates in numerous speaking engagements and presentations to a variety of audiences worldwide.

Chapter 1
Collision of Contexts and Conscience

This chapter provides an overview and global introduction to the content. In the introduction, understanding of core concepts of public health, equity, justice, and health are established. This chapter centers on unpacking the meaning of health, how health is understood and misunderstood, and most importantly how health is created. Its impact in producing outcomes across the determinants of health is examined across an ecological spectrum of the populations, communities, and the system of care. The conceptual exploration of just health and what the creation of a more just system of health means is introduced and situated in relation to our society and why health matters.

1.1 Introduction

The context of health as we know it has been filtered through many variations of descriptions and lenses. Often health is thought of in relation to physical wellness and prioritized accordingly. Health has been considered as a state where disease is absent, which is believed to be indicative of being healthy. As providers of "health," we align our provision of health services with this fundamental belief of what health is and by default what it is not. All of this occurs within systems that too have defined health in ways that are congruent with this fundamental belief that health is primarily about the absence of disease. So, we begin with defining health as it has traditionally been understood or misunderstood, and potentially how it can be reimagined. Situating the historical and current discourse of health is critical to understanding the reimagining of health toward justice in health. It's a leap to connect justice and health without a clear understanding of either and arguing their interrelatedness. To do this, we have to explore not just the definitions of health but also our fundamental beliefs about health.

As a society, we have our own values and assumptions about what we do and do not believe health is. Likewise, as providers we also show up with our own values

C. Burnett, *Justice in Health*, https://doi.org/10.1007/978-3-031-18504-5_1

and assumptions about health that might be reflective of or divergent from the over-all beliefs of our society. Where the ideas and values of our society and those of the individual converge is the starting point of reference for our understanding of health and our beliefs of what it is.

One of the most undervalued and underdeveloped explorations in my opinion is the examination of health; what it means and what belief systems are embedded in those definitions. This requires the critical analysis of both the definitions and the discourses of health. Without the intentional unpacking of these narratives about health, we limit the exploration of the full spectrum of its possibilities and opportu-nities. Most important to this process are the potential impacts and opportunities a refreshed view of health creates for our system of health care, our providers, and populations, specifically those bearing the brunt of health disparities.

Examining the narratives of health is a critical starting point to engage with and fully examine the discourse of health. Here we can identify what it means to be healthy and move toward recalibrating health in a way that advocates for creating health through justice. Health narratives connect the discourse of health with the ideology that shapes it which can solidify our understanding of why the connection with health and justice matter and need to be made. This is an attempt to process and repurpose health more inclusively. Stripping down our definition, narratives, and beliefs about health will enable us to consume a new construction of health that sits within the gradient of justice.

1.2 Historical Pathways to Defining Health

The World Health Organization (WHO) believes in health as a fundamental princi-ple embedded with its constitution where health is defined as "a state of complete physical, mental and social well-being and not merely the absence of disease or infirmity" (https://www.who.int/about/governance/constitution). Adopted in early 1946, this constitution was the outcome of the international health conference, con-vened to establish a global health agency endorsed by 61 states. Member States, in principle, not only agreed with the definition of health but also understood the func-tion of health to include "the enjoyment of which should be part of the rightful heri-tage of " every human being without distinction of race, religion, political belief, economic or social condition" (WHO Official Records, 1946, p. 16). President Truman opened the first meeting of the international health conference on June 19, 1946, acknowledging the devastating impacts of the recent war in exacerbating health issues and destroying the health infrastructure. He applauded the formation of this new health organization as a mechanism for global coordination and strength-ening of health (WHO Official Records, 1946, p. 31) and resolved that:

> The right to adequate medical care and the opportunity to achieve and enjoy good health should be available to all people. For this objective I can assure you of the interest and the support of the United States. (WHO Official Records, 1946, p. 31)

The historical text from the formation of the World Health Organization demonstrates two critical fundamental principles of the definition of health. The first being that health is viewed as a required societal asset to human progress and that its access is an essential human right. Health is viewed as both a value and a condition of person and community. Two years following the formation of the World Health Organization, the United Nations General Assembly adopted the Universal Declaration of Human Rights (UDHR) (https://www.un.org/en/universal-declaration-human-rights). This declaration codified 30 articles of inalienable human rights protections, one being article 25, that directly addresses health. Article 25 of the UNDHR states that:

(1) Everyone has the right to a standard of living adequate for the health and well-being of himself and of his family, including food, clothing, housing and medical care and necessary social services, and the right to security in the event of unemployment, sickness, disability, widowhood, old age or other lack of livelihood in circumstances beyond his control. (https://www.un.org/en/universal-declaration-human-rights)

Within both foundational health defining documents are their common threading of health as more than the absence of disease and the status of health as a right. The crux of these notions paves the pathway for defining health and serves to identify where along the spectrum of these definitions that our current structures, systems, and practice function. Moreover, these two health spaces also illuminate the degree to which we have internalized and operationalized health as either a right (or not) or as simply disease absence or presence. Both determine the point of departure for our actions, inactions, decisions, and health consequences. It is important to point out that the United States along with several other countries are signatories to both documents which should in theory attest to a commitment and endorsement of such ideals. Yet in application, we see many examples of disconnect and misalignment with our health beliefs and those as outlined by the World Health Organization and within the Universal Declaration of Human Rights.

Dialogue and discourse are shaped by context and have to be understood as a part of the context in which they are located. There is an interdiscursiveness of the dialectic that positions context in relation to how it is experienced and translated by and through words. What makes our understanding of these pivotal definitions of health most intriguing is knowing what occurred during and around the inception of both documents that (a) became the impetus for their creation and (b) informed the ideas and choice of language. The formation of the World Health Organization and the creation of the United Nations Declaration of Human Rights came on the heels of a global traumatic event: World War II. World War II which lasted between 1939 and 1945 is believed to have been the deadliest war of all time involving 30 countries at a cost of over 70 million lives (the impact of WWII) (Amadeo, 2021). During this time, the world experienced unimaginable famine, poverty, disease, death, and despair. Fear, grief, uncertainty, and hopelessness were ever present for many countries and populations under and engaged in attack. The war had torn and decimated the deepest human, moral, and social fabric of many societies and dissolved their sense of peace and security. It created enormous and far-reaching economic, physical, and psychological consequences transforming beliefs and values around many ideals including health. Several post-WWII acts such as the formation of the United Nations (https://www.un.org/en/about-us/history-of-the-un), the North Atlantic Treaty Organization (NATO) (https://www.nato.int/nato-welcome/index.html), the General Agreement on Tariffs and Trade and subsequent World Trade Organization (https://www.wto.org/english/thewto_e/history_e/history_e.htm), and the Council of Europe (a precursor to the European Union) (https://www.coe.int/en/web/about-us/founding-fathers) each emerged from the desolation and liberation of the war. These exemplars attest to the nature of context in shaping beliefs and values that then translate to action. The world desperately needed leadership toward a more humane and peaceful future that was inextricably tied to the health of many nations, and the WHO and UNDHR were part of the critical response.

Moments in time matter and inform our health beliefs and the value we place on health. The COVID-19 pandemic (https://www.cdc.gov/coronavirus/2019-nCoV/) has been one such pivotal moment in time, full of tension, polarization, and resistance around global health and health policy, the health of nations, and in particular, the health crises of disparate populations. It has caused us to question not only the definition of health but the equity and justice of health. These positions and orientations extend consideration of the person's context and that of the entire health workforce. Arguably there has not been a time in modern history where the right to health and health as a human right have collided more traumatically and urgently than during COVID-19. This collision of health "rights" is the transformative opportunity to rethink not only our long-standing definitions of health but also transform the beliefs accompanying those definitions. Defining health outside of the pathological means redefining it inclusive of the contextual influences and disparities that shape it. Reconstructing conceptions of health and specifically justice in health factors in the unseen and insidious drivers of health such as racism, equity, power, and oppression. We attempt a more consolidated and humanizing definition of health built on the examination of the existent definitions of health such as a resource for everyday living (The Ottawa Charter for Health Promotion, 1986); human flourishing (Card, 2019); and Dietrich Bonhoeffer definitions of health as "the strength to be" (Missilbrook, 2014).

1.2.1 Health as a Resource for Everyday Living

Health as a resource for everyday living was first introduced in 1986 at the International Conference on Health Promotion which enshrined the Ottawa Charter (The Ottawa Charter for Health Promotion, 1986). Within this Charter (see full-text: Appendix A), the resource of health is a social and individual responsibility, determined by several prerequisites that are influenced by political, economic, social, cultural, environmental, behavioral, and biological conditions (The Ottawa Charter for Health Promotion, 1986). The Charter's inception was precipitated by the global desire to achieve health for all by the year 2000. It was a commitment to promote health, advocate for health equity, to close health gaps and elevate the belief in health as a large-scale social investment. Health as a resource introduces resource terminology into the human domain, which is a far cry from the more common framing of "resource" used in discussions of finance and economy. From that perspective, resources imply commodification, allocation, and capitalization. When juxtaposed within the dominion of health, our understanding of health encompasses a measured quantity that needs to be balanced somewhere between replenishment and monitoring.

Williamson and Carr (2009) conceptual exploration of health as a resource illuminates the challenges in understanding "health as capital." They assert that failing to contemplate health as a resource has implications for policy and practice that have yet to be examined. While they posit the meaning of health as a resource for everyday living to be somewhat elusive to those who are expected to uphold it, more problematic is the application of this definition. At issue is really the commodification of health without a clear understanding and implications of health as a commodity. For example, health as capital does imply investment which by nature of economic association should provide a "return." Several unknowns exist on both the investment and the return sides to exploring health as capital. On the investment end, an unquantified amount of "health capital" is assumed to be available equitably to any individual for the subsequent investment into themselves to the benefit of the person and society at large. There is no clearly articulated starting point for the acquisition of health and no identified quantity which earmarks the beginning of "health" or level of sufficient. The points as to "how" health starts and from "where" it starts and "how" it is equitably attained or sustained are missing.

As with any traded commodity, there are an explicitly assigned value (starting point), a designated location for gaining entry (markets, brokers), and the ability to view and monitor both. Within a commodities orientation to health, the commodity (health) is not laid out. With no indication of its starting value or starting location, this creates a messy baseline measure for establishing a definition and meaning. Additionally, there is a failure to factor in the variation in positionality of the individual in relation to their well-being and access to controls for improving their overall health. If health is a resource, we must understand the location of the individual in relation to the resource and the ability of the individual to obtain the resource. The location of the individual is not in reference to their physical health status, but rather their prerequisite status for being able to obtain health and what health uniquely means to them and their context. At the other end of the spectrum of the health commodities orientation is the premise of a "return." As a resource, the presumed health return happens to both the individual and society. Yet the extent and success of this return is difficult to objectively discern, especially in the space of determining what is an equitable and just return.

Extenuating factors that mitigate and/or moderate health as a resource are drivers to be considered within the definition of health as a resource for everyday living and not external to it. So while this definition has been widely accepted as a more progressive definition of health, it does miss critical essentials that would deepen and clarify its definition. Therefore, from this standpoint, health becomes challenging to practically apply in practice and policy creating gaps and inconsistencies in actualizing this concept.

1.2.2   Health as a by-Product of Health Promotion

Health promotion is viewed as a key instrument of action to achieving health as a resource for everyday living. Within the Ottawa Charter (1986), the role of health promotion is delineated around essential spaces where health work is needed and necessary to ensure health. What followed 10 years later was the Jakarta Declaration[10] (1998) (see Appendix B for full text), intended to strengthen the view of health promotion as a facilitator to the development of health. The Jakarta Declaration (1997) identified core strategies built on those identified in the Ottawa Charter (1986) to further encourage comprehensive and integrated approaches to health promotion. Poverty is stated as the greatest threat to the attainment of health and attending to new health challenges of mental health, infectious disease, demographic trends, and transnational influencers of health are the prioritized action points for health promotion (https://scielosp.org/pdf/rpsp/1998.v3n1/58-61/en). Importantly, in Jakarta Declaration (1997), the social determinants of health are identified as prerequisites for health that require an evolved approach to health promotion to address them which is the impetus for a stated call to action to create a global alliance for health promotion. The alliance function is to advance several outlined key health promotion priorities outlined to tackle the emerging health threats and strengthen health into the twenty-first century.

Within the almost 10-year span between the Ottawa Charter (1986) and Jakarta Declaration (1997), a pronounced sense of increasing global urgency to address "health" more broadly with a heightened focus on health promotion as the solution for mitigating obstacles to achieving "health" is evident. Beyond the Jakarta Declaration (1997) statement that health is "a basic human right" which is "essential for social and economic development," a full exploration of this definition is not offered. Less clear is how can we mobilize equitable and just global support of health promotion in the obvious absence of an explicit definition of what health is and what health at a population level would mean within the expected call to action? Additionally, where are the social determinants of health situated within the spectrum of defining health if it is viewed as a prerequisite to health and not an embodiment of health? Sorting out such nuances of the definition of health is important to not only the implementation of health promotion activities that the global community is being asked to address "with urgency" but also in determining what successful outcomes or achievement of outcomes look like. Measuring our achievement in health promotion becomes difficult without clearly defined targets of "health" success. If we are unclear about what "health" is, then we are unable with any real certainty to identify our achievement of it and accountability for it.

1.3   The Social Determinants of Health as Health

Globally, we fell far too short of our well-intended efforts toward the achievement for Health for All by 2000. On the rise and gaining momentum during this milestone era was the pivot toward health as a right resulting from increasing attention to health inequities and widening health disparities. Smaller international conferences such as the International Society for Equity in Health (ISEqH) Conferences produced the Toronto Declaration on Equity in Health (2002) (https://academic.oup.com/heapro/article/19/2/269/604701), which ignited the call for global action in social determinants of health through equity. At this conference, the goal was to (a) consider the state of ten key social or societal determinants of health across Canada; (b) explore the implications of these conditions for the health of Canadians; and (c) outline policy directions to improve the health of Canadians by influencing the quality of these determinants of health (https://academic.oup.com/heapro/article/19/2/269/604701). Within this Declaration, the identification of health as a human right, ten social determinants of health—early life, education, employment and working conditions, food security, health services, housing, income and income distribution, social exclusion, the social safety net, and unemployment and job insecurity—were selected as influencers of health equity (https://academic.oup.com/heapro/article/19/2/269/604701).

Global interpretations of the term "health" being used along very loosely defined threads were being shifted. Health was now believed to transcend beyond a resource and/or a by-product of promotion. It needed to be recognized as *more* because health disparities and gaps in inequities were rising with rapid persistence.

Political, economic, and social drivers were seen as the core culprits behind this disturbing trend that disproportionately affected racialized communities, women, rural populations, and the poor. Inequities and the conditions that create them catalyzed support for accepting the social determinants of health as health. The Toronto Declaration on Equity in Health (2002) called on the global community and specifically the World Health Organization, governments, and health professionals to act. Action was requested across sectors, policies, and systems to bolster accountability, investments, and system change in health equity (The Toronto Declaration on Equity in Health, 2002).

This was echoed during the World Conference on Social Determinants of Health in Rio which produced the 2011 Rio Declaration on the Social Determinants of Health (WHO, 2011) (See Appendix C for Full Text). Health, although not defined, is described as "essential to create inclusive, equitable, economically productive and healthy societies" and a key feature "of what constitutes a successful, inclusive and fair society in the 21st century" (WHO, 2011, sect. 6, p. 2). The signatories expressed belief in an "all for equity" approach where the responsibility to create equity belonged to everyone to achieve good health and "good health" "requires a universal, comprehensive, equitable, effective, responsive and accessible quality health system" (WHO, 2011 sect. 7, p. 2).

The momentum around the social determinants of health as an indicator of health grew with and was shaped by the swelling tide advocating for the advancement of sustainable development. According to the United Nations, sustainable development "meets the needs of the present without compromising the ability of future generations to meet their own needs" and consists of economic development, social development, and environmental protection (United Nations, n.d.). At its core, sustainable development's ultimate aim is the eradication of poverty by focusing on equitable economic and social development and ecological conservation. The

United Nations 2012 Future We Want Resolution (United Nations General Assembly, 2012) readily moved sustainable development to an accelerated priority agenda item in recognition that fundamentally over the previous 20 years little had changed for the majority of the impoverished world, in fact it had gotten worse.

> We are deeply concerned that one in five people on this planet, or over 1 billion people, still live in extreme poverty, and that one in seven or 14 percent is undernourished, while public health challenges, including pandemics and epidemics, remain omnipresent threats. In this context, we note the ongoing discussions on human security in the General Assembly. We acknowledge that with the world's population projected to exceed 9 billion by 2050 with an estimated two thirds living in cities, we need to increase our efforts to achieve sustainable development and, in particular, the eradication of poverty, hunger and preventable diseases (United Nations General Assembly, 2012, Res 66/288, Sect 21.)

Human security is needed to achieve sustainable development and sustainable development cannot be achieved without human security. To pursue human security, we have to interpret health within the sphere of an emerging sustainable development agenda. Creating a global agenda means that first, existing systems need to be strengthened and coordinated across structures, government, and industry to achieve the global sustainable development agenda; and every institution and sector must play an active role in achieving "success" of this agenda. Social, economic, and environmental determinants are integrated influences of human security which in turn influence the sustainable development agenda. What this resolution helped to articulate was a deep reaffirmation of human rights and its connectedness with health from the lens of sustainable development. It provided another pathway for thinking about health within the construct of human rights to achieve social equity necessary for optimal sustainable development.

1.4   The Rights of Health

Health and human rights are fairly aligned in their quest to center the equal treatment of all human beings. Arguably these rights could be perceived as one in the same yet consensus in support of human rights is more likely than the support of health as a right. When extending health as a human right with an afforded inherent right to health, rationalizations and polarization as to why this should or should not happen occur. Nowhere is this more passionately debated than in the United States, where sentiments of the right to health are viewed with suspicion as a currency of socialism. Fear of big government and the overreach of government is part of the slippery slope that fuels this suspicion and the reluctance to embrace the right to health for all. Ideology surrounding the right to health as socialism incognito and health as a right as aligned with human rights are two profound points of departure that warrant the need to unpack the definition of health.

Earlier in this chapter, you were introduced to the UN Declaration on Human Rights. Enshrined within that declaration is the acknowledgment and endorsement of the right to health. Many other international rights declarations ratified by countries around the world such as the International Covenant on Economic, Social, and Cultural Rights (ICESCR), the Convention on the Rights of the Child (CRC), and the International Convention on the Elimination of All Forms of Racial Discrimination *health* positioned as *the right to health* is tacitly threaded throughout (Blackman et al., 2008). Health as a human right has been explicitly identified by the World Health Organization which according to their Health as Human Rights Fact Sheet (2017) (Appendix D) is reiterated in their 1946 Constitution and entails principles, elements, and components of health understood as an obligatory human right (https://www.who.int/news-room/fact-sheets/detail/human-rights-and-health). The World Health Organization (2017) contends that:

> The right to the highest attainable standard of health" implies a clear set of legal obligations on states to ensure appropriate conditions for the enjoyment of health for all people without discrimination. The right to health is one of a set of internationally agreed human rights standards, and is inseparable or 'indivisible' from these other rights. This means achieving the right to health is both central to, and dependent upon, the realisation of other human rights, to food, housing, work, education, information, and participation (https://www.who.int/news-room/fact-sheets/detail/human-rights-and-health).

These are positions that while endorsed have yet to be fully embraced nor implemented across health systems and health practices in the United States.

In part, building consensus around what exactly a right to health means and what claiming the right health looks like across populations, systems, and in practice has been problematic. Populations facing the most health disparities are in desperate need of health as a humanistic right. To believe in health as a right account is to believe that every human being regardless of status, race, or location has the inherent right to a healthful life. What a life full of health and one unbridled with the capacity to achieve health looks like will vary across many axes of person, family, culture, and societies. The social and built environment needed to procure a healthful life is also essential to constructing a definition of health within a rights framework. Factors such as race, ethnicity, gender, social location, geography, wealth, opportunity, neighborhoods, and employment create conditions that affect the achievement of health as a right. The right-to-health perspective forcefully engages the narrative of access into its definition. Access to health services, innovation, and opportunity are essential components that shape the right to health. Together health as a right (statement of what it is) and the right to health (statement of advocacy to obtain health) merge to formulate an action orientated definition of health that embeds the principle of rights.

Health systems are a critical part of the solution arm for the application of health as a right. For the most part, health systems are predominantly thought of within a tertiary orientation. When we think of a healthcare system, highest on the list are hospitals and clinics. Much lower are community spaces (schools, churches, non-medical agencies, homecare) and until the COVID-19 pandemic, public health. Dominant actors of the healthcare system include the healthcare system, health insurance companies, government health policies (Medicaid/Medicare/health exchanges), and actual healthcare providers. The focus is on downstream approaches such as treatment, medical interventions, disease outbreaks, and "sickcare" and less on upstream (prevention, early intervention, conditions, and root causes of health). The "system" in its hyper-downstream focus and current siloed configuration of offerings against a backdrop of profit and non-profit facilitators do influence access and create barriers that are not conducive to supporting a health rights orientation. In fact, it's just the opposite.

There is a disconnect between this definition of health and its application within the dominant system and by the brokers of health themselves. The system as we know it cannot provide rights it was never designed to create. For health rights to be taken up in earnest, it must attend to those aspects which implement and sustain those rights; otherwise, it is another aspirational definition only achievable if all other conditions work accordingly. Otherwise, the right to health will remain beyond the purview of the individual who needs it the most which brings its definitional appropriateness into question. It also calls into question the responsibility for the provision of those rights and what a sufficient "measure" of health rights should look like across populations, communities, and systems. In essence, what and where is the threshold of accountability by which these rights are actualized?

1.5   Health as a Right in Practice

Convergence around the definition of health and the structures needed to build it occur in the delivery of health defined as a right. As healthcare providers, there is a taken for granted assumption in our inherent belief in health as a right. The condition of health develops in stages which vary based on conditions external to the individual. As providers predominately trained within structures and institutions that react to health, we are not incentivized to practice in a health rights framework or educated within an orientation that focuses on operationalizing this definition of health. Yet ultimately, we are assumed to be capable of providing "it." I first encountered this dose of reality teaching a health policy course to graduate health professional students, many of whom were already engaged in practice. When pressed about the notion of health as a right, it was perceived by close to a 1/3 of that class as *radical*. So how do we reconcile the belief of health, if defined as a right, within our practice if those who already believe in health are pressed to make this most obvious of connections?

Adopting health as a right into practice introduces the healthcare system into the context. We are training healthcare providers within a system that does not operationally support a definition of health as a right. Boldly speaking, one would be stretched to identify how health systems define health as a right and what would be accepted as a definitive demonstration of achieving health? Is that discharge from the hospital? Is it recovery from sickness? Is it managing chronic disease? What exactly does health as a right look like within the current system of care and to the providers within that system who are providing health support to families, clients, and communities toward being healthy?

It feels like a moving target that sounds ideal but that has not been universally implemented or practiced consistently. If the right to health were to be the assumed defining parameters to achieve health, then how might that look in practice? At what point or better yet what is the threshold for knowing that we have achieved health defined as a right? What does the appropriate measure of health rights look like and for whom—does this differ from population to population based on extent of disparity or is health as a right doled out in equal measure because the notion of rights implies equality versus equity? Can or should the right to health be premised on equality or equity? Health defined as right in theory sounds good; however, in practice, it is under-developed and less optimized in health spaces where access to those same spaces are not based on universal right of all to have health. Until these and many of the other questions raised are answered, it is difficult to determine if this definition of health is one that truly captures the essence of whatever it is seeking. It feels like a premature leap that oversteps fundamental questions of practice, structures, and accountability and lacks clarity in the role that context, location, and intersectional experiences play in being able to access health as a right. It leans toward an exchange of the commodity of health which in and of itself is not well understood. While there is a deep appreciation for defining health as right; in some respects, it does not go far enough in capturing a universal understanding of what health is and as a result knowing that we have achieved it.

1.6   Just Health (Justice in Health)

Just health is defined as the strength to obtain and achieve human flourishing through just and equitable health systems, structures, and practices that are co-created and co-informed by health narratives and needs of the individual and the context of the community. It allows for the establishment of health sovereignty where the understanding of health is infused with cultural humility, historical knowing, and the acquisition of health assets to produce responsive outcomes that maximize well-being.

Shifting our attention to the definition of health as justice is a process of emancipatory knowing that (a) centers the meaning of health in a more democratized way to capture and prioritize the needs of individual within and informed by their context; (b) emboldens the systems to structurally attend to the conditions that shape health; and (c) clearly assigns a solution and an impact lens to achieving health beyond the limitations of the most current paradigms of health. It requires three essential elements: emancipatory knowing, structural justice, and sovereignty.

Emancipatory knowing helps us to understand health justice by forcing the critical examination and understanding of root issues, systems of oppression, and conditions that impact individuals, communities, and society. The illumination from this examination is what creates emancipation in knowledge. Structural justice posits that rectifying inequity in structures, outcomes, and opportunity are essential to achieving health. Sovereignty embeds the democratization and co-creation of health with the expected outcome of human flourishing. We will examine each of these essential elements more deeply.

Any arrogance and ignorance that would dilute our understanding of justice in health is best counteracted with the basic philosophical premise of emancipatory knowing. Emancipatory knowledge is rooted in the critical paradigm engaging consciousness, reflexivity, and the analysis of power that situates many theories including critical race, postcolonial, post structural, and intersectionality (Wesp et al., 2018).

Healthcare professionals for the most part have not widely engaged in the uptake of this paradigm to inform their practice and research. In general, the individual and more importantly the health of the individual is understood in a manner that is decontextualized from their environment, their community, and society at large. Or the social determinants of health are introduced as important health considerations with abstraction about how and why they came to be a determining factor in one's health. With ever-increasing disparities and inequities in the most marginalized of populations, we have seen critical nursing scholars embrace this orientation to guide and inform their work. In 2000, Cowling et al. (2000) published the highly influential nursing manifesto which critiqued and challenges current healthcare practices by squarely calling for humanizing and social justice infusion of nursing practice that (a) values experiential elements health and wellness and (b) "no longer consider our values and actions out of the context of all beings" (Cowling et al., 2000, section II.a)[17]. According to Kagan et al. (2010), the manifesto:

> …indicates concern about an over-emphasis in nursing on specialization, disembodied physiology, and diagnosis and treatment. The authors of the Manifesto embrace unitary and wholeness perspectives because within the theoretical basis is that belief that there is no separation between humans and the environment. While others may not agree, this viewpoint is considered optimal because it suggests an inclusivity and connection that easily underpins a social justice framework for solving the problems of humans and the environment. To some, this is precisely the standpoint from which to effect meaningful social or disciplinary change (Kagan et al., 2010, p. 80).

Embracing this orientation endorses the belief that social structures create, drive and diminish health and therefore nurses and other providers of health are obligated to initiate and lead conscious action to produce transformative change through emancipatory knowing. Emancipatory knowing occurs when hidden realities of oppression and power of societal conditions and structures are revealed and the knower becomes enlightened by this new knowledge which extends beyond the dominant discourse and embraces multiple ways of knowing (Browne, 2000). Ultimately when knowledge of hidden realities and oppressive conditions of beings are moved into the realm of one's consciousness, this propels the knower toward action. You cannot have action without this shift in consciousness which prioritizes the context of the human experience as an interconnected phenomenon of being and central to one's health.

1.6.1   Understanding Justice in Health Within Structural Justice

It is important to understand that beyond context, community, and individuals, health occurs within and is created by structures. Any reforms to health and well-being must engage in structural atonement of structural conditions such as policies, procedure and resources, and system "actors" that determine and undermine health. Defining health within a structural orientation identifies the interconnectedness of structures as an essential component of health.

Structural justice frames the need for equity, humanity, and synergy to be an integral part of structures at the onset to achieve optimal outcomes. This means we must disrupt and illuminate structural impediments to human dignity in order to intentionally redress inequity and create human flourishing. At its core, this is what structural justice is and what it must entail. By definition, structural justice "acknowledges the oppressive and re-victimizing inherent nature of structures as unacceptable and requires purposeful rectification. It demands that primacy and privilege be extended to the most vulnerable, through sustainable structural processes that attend to equity, power and human dignity" (Burnett et al., 2018, p. 11). Attending to intentional structural reconciliation is to truly understanding health in the most inclusive and encompassing way. It is a necessary act of goodwill and trust that is paramount to creating health particularly in communities where there is historical mistrust specific to healthcare providers and of systems and institutions that have perpetuated disparities and inequity.

Structural justice is the accountability framework to bridge the gap between health equities and disparities which makes it a key animator of health. Considering justice in health is to examine and rectify the structural engines and systems that shape health. We have seen the consequences of not addressing systemic inequity, the most obvious being perpetual health disparities and diminishing health outcomes that affect the most vulnerable of populations. Without the transformation of structures, a critical element of root causes is overlooked. Structural justice demands the structural contextualization of health as a means of understanding the conditions that influence and compromise health in order to fix them. It is the bridging of the ontological and empirical toward a pathway where knowledge about structural drivers of health is funneled into action for flourishing of individuals, communities, and our society.

1.6.2   Understanding Justice in Health Within Sovereignty

Creating sovereignty in health is a process of deconstructing health narratives to reconstruct a self-determined meaning of health that accentuates assets, strengths, and culture. It is co-created and co-informed to reflect a tailored outcome that represents human flourishing. Ultimately health sovereignty is the culmination of all the defined and undefined parameters of health that affect the human condition in relation to a person's context and environment, freeing one to be healthy in a way that honors resilience, culture, and situatedness. It is strengths-based and culturally humble. Being sovereign in one's health is to encompass autonomous flourishing based on the subjective account of the lived life that include both outcomes and states of being. It is radically inclusive and human-centered as informed by expertise of the person, community, and context. At the most basic of levels, pathways to human flourishing entail equitable access to satisfaction and joy in life; access to opportunity and innovation; embodied mental and physical health; attaining meaning and purpose; and having character, virtue, and close social relationships (Vanderweele, 2017) in a sustained and stable way. Creating a sustained and stable environment requires inputs (resources) and influencers (ecological context) of human flourishing which occur along an intersectional and symbiotic trajectory. According to Bunker (2010), "human flourishing can prosper when empathy, compassion, and solidarity are lived in communion with others" (Bunker, 2010, p. 292). Hence all facets of human liberation and dignity must be in alignment to achieve sovereignty in health.

Another consideration for defining health within a lens of sovereignty is believing in health as the *strength to be*. The concept of health as a *strength to be* is one that liberates us from the traditional confines of health within a biomedical model to one that embraces positive outlooks on health from the individuals' perspective (Misselbrook, 2014). With this understanding comes the important shift of defining health to conceptualizing health, thus allowing for fluidity of experiences, interpretation, and diverse health identities. Huber et al. (2011) propose that the concept of health to be formulated within an adaptive and self-managed space "regarded as a dynamic balance between opportunities and limitations, shifting through life and affected by external conditions such as social and environmental challenges" (Huber et al., 2011, p. 2). Loosening the confining existing health definitions toward the justice in health elements we have been discussing allows for infusion of critical health drivers within a human-centered approach as central enablers of the discourse.

1.7 Culture and Health

Often overlooked is the recognition that for centuries, cultures have embedded health traditions that have been excluded from the current Western-centered health narratives and practices. Our pursuit to understand and conceptualize health is premised upon the belief that health is more richly informed by embracing cultural narratives of health and the inclusion of other health traditions and practices. Moreover, we experience health and its impacts globally and locally with the reality that many diverse populations and ethnic groups exposure to "typical" health services, support, and delivery of care are culturally shaped and informed. Williams and Mikola (2018) highlight superdiversity viewed as a complex intersectional ecosystem of culture, ethnicity, context, and experiences which require dynamic adaptation of systems to meet uniquely personal trajectories. For these and other reasons, this ecosystem shapes health outcomes and disparities quite visibly along lines of race, ethnicity, and culture. While we are aware of the negative health sequelae pervasive in diverse populations, less often are we exposed to facilitators of health that foster resilience and hope. These are deeply situated in a spectrum of cultural health traditions the breadth of which is not possible to cover in this section. Still, it is necessary to elevate the impact of culture, cultural belief, and practices within a justice in health orientation. Indigenous, First Nations, and native people around the world have used various mediums for conveying and manifesting health which is determined within their own traditions and narratives.

Much of those narratives are restorative in nature often laden with stories and practices that highlight autonomy, hope, and resilience. Blix et al. (2012) adopt the understanding of health not only as a subjective experience but where stories are critical to examining health insights from an integrated embodied perspective which centers agency and context. They used this approach to study the health narratives of the Sami indigenous people of Norway which they found demonstrated active resilience and revealed "untold" truths that illuminated Sami health processes. Narratives of health in the African American community are examined by Davis (2013) who discovered that health is created by community and individual empowerment through transformative innovation that happens within spaces of storytelling, healing rituals, and social practices. Health converges in performance (the doing) and through a spiritual cuisine "a metaphorical description of the relational and interactive patterns of people, health discourse, and cultural expression that intermingle" (Davis, 2013, p. 144) in communal space. Understanding health among diverse populations is to know that it is experienced in moments of strength and resilience and not just within the constructed narrative of pathology, victimization, and disparity (Hatala et al., 2016).

1.8   Conclusion

Health is a term with an evolving definition that should be revisited to align its interpretation to meet the current context. What this chapter has shown is the limitations of the current definitions of health to meet the needs and issues of now and where lies the opportunities for advancing how we view and define the meaning of health. Justice in health—Just health—is meant to democratize the playing field of health starting with its definition. It allows for the deconstruction of antiquated definitions of health toward a more transformative definition of health—where health is reframed, reimagined, and reprioritized beyond a static state or destination. Health is fluid and in the moment as are our ways of knowing about health and being healthy. Justice in Health advances the historical health narrative to understanding health through emancipatory knowing, structural justice, and sovereignty which creates a health ecosystem where health solutions are inherently and proactively responsive to the individual, community, and the context.

1.9   Reflective Questions and Considerations

1. How have you conceptualized health and how is it similar to or different from Justice in Health?
2. What ways can the United States use the ratified international charters to inform and reform the current system of care?
3. Should health be considered a right? Unpack and explain how it can be ensured if it is, and if it is not, a right then what should it be considered?

Appendices

Appendix A: Ottawa Charter for Health Promotion, 1986[1]

Health Promotion

Health promotion is the process of enabling people to increase control over, and to improve, their health. To reach a state of complete physical mental and social well-being, an individual or group must be able to identify and to realize aspirations, to satisfy needs, and to change or cope with the environment. Health is, therefore, seen as a resource for everyday life, not the objective of living. Health is a positive concept emphasizing social and personal resources, as well as physical capacities. Therefore, health promotion is not just the responsibility of the health sector but goes beyond healthy lifestyles to well-being.

Prerequisites for Health

The fundamental conditions and resources for health are peace, shelter, education, food, income, a stable ecosystem, sustainable resources, social justice, and equity. Improvement in health requires a secure foundation in these basic prerequisites.

Advocate

Good health is a major resource for social, economic, and personal development and an important dimension of quality of life. Political, economic, social, cultural, environmental, behavioral, and biological factors can all favor health or be harmful

---

[1] Reprinted from *Ottawa Charter for Health Promotion, 1986*, World Health Organization/Europe, Copyright 1986. https://www.euro.who.int/__data/assets/pdf_file/0004/129532/Ottawa_Charter. pdf. Accessed on August 3, 2022.

to it. Health promotion action aims at making these conditions favorable through advocacy for health.

Enable

Health promotion focuses on achieving equity in health. Health promotion action aims at reducing differences in current health status and ensuring equal opportunities and resources to enable all people to achieve their fullest health potential. This includes a secure foundation in a supportive environment, access to information, life skills, and opportunities for making healthy choices. People cannot achieve their fullest health potential unless they are able to take control of those things which determine their health. This must apply equally to women and men.

Mediate

The prerequisites and prospects for health cannot be ensured by the health sector alone. More importantly, health promotion demands coordinated action by all concerned: by governments, by health and other social and economic sectors, by non-governmental and voluntary organizations, by local authorities, by industry, and by the media. People in all walks of life are involved as individuals, families, and communities. Professional and social groups and health personnel have a major responsibility to mediate between differing interests in society for the pursuit of health.

Health promotion strategies and programs should be adapted to the local needs and possibilities of individual countries and regions to take into account differing social, cultural, and economic systems.

Health Promotion Action Means

Build Healthy Public Policy

Health promotion goes beyond health care. It puts health on the agenda of policy-makers in all sectors and at all levels, directing them to be aware of the health consequences of their decisions and to accept their responsibilities for health.

Health promotion policy combines diverse but complementary approaches including legislation, fiscal measures, taxation, and organizational change. It is coordinated action that leads to health, income, and social policies that foster greater equity. Joint action contributes to ensuring safer and healthier goods and services, healthier public services, and cleaner, more enjoyable environments.

Health promotion policy requires the identification of obstacles to the adoption of healthy public policies in non-health sectors and ways of removing them. The aim must be to make the healthier choice the easier choice for policy-makers as well.

Create Supportive Environments

Our societies are complex and interrelated. Health cannot be separated from other goals. The inextricable links between people and their environment constitute the basis for a socioecological approach to health. The overall guiding principle for the world, nations, regions, and communities alike is the need to encourage reciprocal maintenance—to take care of each other, our communities, and our natural environment. The conservation of natural resources throughout the world should be emphasized as a global responsibility.

Changing patterns of life, work, and leisure have a significant impact on health. Work and leisure should be a source of health for people. The way society organizes work should help create a healthy society. Health promotion generates living and working conditions that are safe, stimulating, satisfying, and enjoyable.

Systematic assessment of the health impact of a rapidly changing environment—particularly in areas of technology, work, energy production, and urbanization—is essential and must be followed by action to ensure positive benefit to the health of the public. The protection of the natural and built environments and the conservation of natural resources must be addressed in any health promotion strategy.

Strengthen Community Action

Health promotion works through concrete and effective community action in setting priorities, making decisions, planning strategies, and implementing them to achieve better health. At the heart of this process is the empowerment of communities, their ownership, and control of their own endeavors and destinies.

Community development draws on existing human and material resources in the community to enhance self-help and social support and to develop flexible systems for strengthening public participation and direction of health matters. This requires full and continuous access to information, learning opportunities for health, as well as funding support.

Develop Personal Skills

Health promotion supports personal and social development through providing information, education for health, and enhancing life skills. By so doing, it increases the options available to people to exercise more control over their own health and over their environments and to make choices conducive to health.

Enabling people to learn throughout life, to prepare themselves for all of its stages, and to cope with chronic illness and injuries is essential. This has to be facilitated in school, home, work, and community settings. Action is required through educational, professional, commercial, and voluntary bodies and within the institutions themselves.

Reorient Health Services

The responsibility for health promotion in health services is shared among individuals, community groups, health professionals, health service institutions, and governments. They must work together toward a healthcare system which contributes to the pursuit of health.

The role of the health sector must move increasingly in a health promotion direction, beyond its responsibility for providing clinical and curative services. Health services need to embrace an expanded mandate which is sensitive and respects cultural needs. This mandate should support the needs of individuals and communities for a healthier life and open channels between the health sector and broader social, political, economic, and physical environmental components.

Reorienting health services also requires stronger attention to health research as well as changes in professional education and training. This must lead to a change of attitude and organization of health services, which refocuses on the total needs of the individual as a whole person.

Moving into the Future

Health is created and lived by people within the settings of their everyday life; where they learn, work, play, and love. Health is created by caring for oneself and others, by being able to take decisions and have control over one's life circumstances, and by ensuring that the society one lives in creates conditions that allow the attainment of health by all its members.

Caring, holism, and ecology are essential issues in developing strategies for health promotion. Therefore, those involved should take as a guiding principle that, in each phase of planning, implementation, and evaluation of health promotion activities, women and men should become equal partners.

Commitment to Health Promotion

The participants in this Conference pledge:

- To move into the arena of healthy public policy, and to advocate a clear political commitment to health and equity in all sectors.
- To counteract the pressures toward harmful products, resource depletion, unhealthy living conditions and environments, and bad nutrition; and to focus attention on public health issues such as pollution, occupational hazards, housing, and settlements.
- To respond to the health gap within and between societies, and to tackle the inequities in health produced by the rules and practices of these societies.
- To acknowledge people as the main health resource; to support and enable them to keep themselves, their families, and friends healthy through financial and

other means; and to accept the community as the essential voice in matters of its health, living conditions, and well-being.
*   To reorient health services and their resources toward the promotion of health; and to share power with other sectors, other disciplines, and most importantly with people themselves.
*   To recognize health and its maintenance as a major social investment and challenge; and to address the overall ecological issue of our ways of living.

The Conference urges all concerned to join them in their commitment to a strong public health alliance.

Call for International Action

The Conference calls on the World Health Organization and other international organizations to advocate the promotion of health in all appropriate forums and to support countries in setting up strategies and programs for health promotion. The Conference is firmly convinced that if people in all walks of life, nongovernmental and voluntary organizations, governments, the World Health Organization, and all other bodies concerned join forces in introducing strategies for health promotion, in line with the moral and social values that form the basis of this Charter, health for all by the year 2000 will become a reality.

Appendix B: Jakarta Declaration on Leading Health Promotion into the Twenty-First Century[2]

The Fourth International Conference on Health Promotion: New Players for a New Era—Leading Health Promotion into the Twenty-First Century, Meeting in Jakarta from 21 to 25 July 1997.

The Fourth International Conference on Health Promotion: New Players for a New Era – Leading Health Promotion into the twenty-first century, meeting in Jakarta from 21 to 25 July 1997, has come at a critical moment in the development of international strategies for health. It is almost 20 years since the World Health Organizations Member States made an ambitious commitment to a global strategy for Health for All and the principles of primary health care through the Declaration of Alma-Ata. It is 11 years since the First International Conference on Health Promotion was held in Ottawa, Canada. That Conference resulted in proclamation of the Ottawa Charter for Health Promotion, which has been a source of guidance and

---

[2] Reproduced from *Jakarta Declaration on Leading Health Promotion into the twenty-first Century*, World Health Organization (WHO), Copyright 1997. https://www.who.int/teams/health-promotion/enhanced-wellbeing/fourth-conference/jakarta-declaration. Accessed on August 3, 2022.

inspiration for health promotion since that time. Subsequent international conferences and meetings have further clarified the relevance and meaning of key strategies in health promotion, including healthy public policy (Adelaide, Australia, 1988), and supportive environments for health (Sundsvall, Sweden, 1991). The Fourth International Conference on Health Promotion is the first to be held in a developing country and the first to involve the private sector in supporting health promotion.

It has provided an opportunity to reflect on what has been learned about effective health promotion, to re-examine the determinants of health, and to identify the directions and strategies that must be adopted to address the challenges of promoting health in the twenty-first century. The participants in the Jakarta Conference hereby present this Declaration on action for health promotion into the next century.

Health Promotion Is a Key Investment

Health is a basic human right and is essential for social and economic development. Increasingly, health promotion is being recognized as an essential element of health development. It is a process of enabling people to increase control over, and to improve, their health. Health promotion, through investment and action, has a marked impact on the determinants of health so as to create the greatest health gain for people, to contribute significantly to the reduction of inequities in health, to further human rights, and to build social capital. The ultimate goal is to increase health expectancy and to narrow the gap in health expectancy between countries and groups.

The Jakarta Declaration on Health Promotion offers a vision and focus for health promotion into the next century. It reflects the firm commitment of participants in the Fourth International Conference on Health Promotion to draw upon the widest possible range of resources to tackle health determinants in the twenty-first century. Determinants of health: new challenges.

The prerequisites for health are peace, shelter, education, social security, social relations, food, income, the empowerment of women, a stable ecosystem, sustainable resource use, social justice, respect for human rights, and equity. Above all, poverty is the greatest threat to health.

Demographic trends such as urbanization, an increase in the number of older people, and the high prevalence of chronic diseases pose new problems in all countries. Other social, behavioral, and biological changes such as increased sedentary behavior, resistance to antibiotics and other commonly available drugs, increased drug abuse, and civil and domestic violence threaten the health and well-being of hundreds of millions of people.

New and re-emerging infectious diseases, and the greater recognition of mental health problems, require an urgent response. It is vital that approaches to health promotion evolve to meet changes in the determinants of health.

Transnational factors also have a significant impact on health. These include the integration of the global economy, financial markets and trade, wide access to media and communications technology, and environmental degradation as a result of the irresponsible use of resources.

These changes shape people's values, their lifestyles throughout the lifespan, and living conditions across the world. Some have great potential for health, such as the development of communications technology, while others, such as international trade in tobacco, have a major negative impact.

Health Promotion Makes a Difference

Research and case studies from around the world provide convincing evidence that health promotion is effective. Health promotion strategies can develop and change lifestyles and have an impact on the social, economic, and environmental conditions that determine health.

Health promotion is a practical approach to achieving greater equity in health. The five strategies set out in the Ottawa Charter for Health Promotion are essential for success:

- Build healthy public policy.
- Create supportive environments.
- Strengthen community action.
- Develop personal skills.
- Reorient health services.

There is now clear evidence that:

- Comprehensive approaches to health development are the most effective. Those that use combinations of the five strategies are more effective than single-track approaches.
- Particular settings offer practical opportunities for the implementation of comprehensive strategies. These include mega-cities, islands, cities, municipalities, local communities, markets, schools, the workplace, and healthcare facilities.
- Participation is essential to sustain efforts. People have to be at the center of health promotion action and decision-making processes for them to be effective.
- health learning fosters participation. Access to education and information is essential to achieving effective participation and the empowerment of people and communities.

These strategies are core elements of health promotion and are relevant for all countries.

New Responses Are Needed

To address emerging threats to health, new forms of action are needed. The challenge for the coming years will be to unlock the potential for health promotion inherent in many sectors of society, among local communities, and within families.

There is a clear need to break through traditional boundaries within government sectors, between governmental and nongovernmental organizations, and between the public and private sectors. Cooperation is essential; this requires the creation of new partnerships for health, on an equal footing, between the different sectors at all levels of governance in societies.

Priorities for Health Promotion in the Twenty-First Century

1. Promote social responsibility for health.
   Decision-makers must be firmly committed to social responsibility. Both the public and private sectors should promote health by pursuing policies and practices that:

   - Avoid harming the health of individuals.
   - Protect the environment and ensure sustainable use of resources.
   - Restrict production of and trade in inherently harmful goods and substances such as tobacco and armaments, as well as discourage unhealthy marketing practices.
   - Safeguard both the citizen in the marketplace and the individual in the workplace.
   - Include equity-focused health impact assessments as an integral part of policy development.

2. Increase investments for health development.

   In many countries, current investment in health is inadequate and often ineffective.
   Increasing investment for health development requires a truly multisectoral approach including, for example, additional resources for education and housing as well as for the health sector.
   Greater investment for health and reorientation of existing investments, both within and among countries, has the potential to achieve significant advances in human development, health, and quality of life.
   Investments for health should reflect the needs of particular groups such as women, children, older people, and Indigenous, poor, and marginalized populations.

3. Consolidate and expand partnerships for health.

   Health promotion requires partnerships for health and social development between the different sectors at all levels of governance and society. Existing partnerships need to be strengthened and the potential for new partnerships must be explored.
   Partnerships offer mutual benefit for health through the sharing of expertise, skills, and resources. Each partnership must be transparent and accountable and be based on agreed ethical principles, mutual understanding, and respect. WHO guidelines should be adhered to.

4. Increase community capacity and empower the individual.

Health promotion is carried out by and with people, not on or to people. It improves both the ability of individuals to take action and the capacity of groups, organizations, or communities to influence the determinants of health.

Improving the capacity of communities for health promotion requires practical education, leadership training, and access to resources. Empowering individuals demands more consistent, reliable access to the decision-making process and the skills and knowledge essential to effect change.

Both traditional communication and the new information media support this process. Social, cultural, and spiritual resources need to be harnessed in innovative ways.

5. Secure an infrastructure for health promotion.

To secure an infrastructure for health promotion, new mechanisms for funding it locally, nationally, and globally must be found. Incentives should be developed to influence the actions of governments, nongovernmental organizations, educational institutions, and the private sector to make sure that resource mobilization for health promotion is maximized. "Settings for health" represent the organizational base of the infrastructure required for health promotion. New health challenges mean that new and diverse networks need to be created to achieve intersectoral collaboration. Such networks should provide mutual assistance within and among countries and facilitate exchange of information on which strategies have proved effective and in which settings.

Training in and practice of local leadership skills should be encouraged in order to support health promotion activities. Documentation of experiences in health promotion through research and project reporting should be enhanced to improve planning, implementation, and evaluation.

All countries should develop the appropriate political, legal, educational, social, and economic environments required to support health promotion.

Call for Action

The participants in this Conference are committed to sharing the key messages of the Jakarta Declaration with their governments, institutions, and communities, putting the actions proposed into practice, and reporting back to the Fifth International Conference on Health Promotion.

In order to speed progress toward global health promotion, the participants endorse the formation of a global health promotion alliance. The goal of this alliance is to advance the priorities for action in health promotion set out in this Declaration.

Priorities for the alliance include:

- Raising awareness of the changing determinants of health.
- Supporting the development of collaboration and networks for health development.

- Mobilizing resources for health promotion.
- Accumulating knowledge on best practice.
- Enabling shared learning.
- Promoting solidarity in action.
- Fostering transparency and public accountability in health promotion.

National governments are called on to take the initiative in fostering and sponsoring networks for health promotion both within and among their countries.

The participants call on the WHO to take the lead in building such a global health promotion alliance and enabling its Member States to implement the outcomes of the Conference. A key part of this role is for the WHO to engage governments, nongovernmental organizations, development banks, organizations of the United Nations system, interregional bodies, bilateral agencies, the labor movement and cooperatives, as well as the private sector, in advancing the priorities for action in health promotion.

Appendix C: Rio Political Declaration on Social Determinants of Health[3]

Rio de Janeiro, Brazil, 21 October 2011.

1. Invited by the World Health Organization, we, Heads of Government, Ministers, and government representatives came together on the 21st day of October 2011 in Rio de Janeiro to express our determination to achieve social and health equity through action on social determinants of health and wellbeing by a comprehensive intersectoral approach.
2. We understand that health equity is a shared responsibility and requires the engagement of all sectors of government, of all segments of society, and of all members of the international community, in an "all for equity" and "health for all" global action.
3. We underscore the principles and provisions set out in the World Health Organization Constitution and in the 1978 Declaration of Alma-Ata as well as in the 1986 Ottawa Charter and in the series of international health promotion conferences, which reaffirmed the essential value of equity in health and recognized that "the enjoyment of the highest attainable standard of health is one of the fundamental rights of every human being without distinction of race, religion, political belief, economic or social condition." We recognize that governments have a responsibility for the health of their peoples, which can be fulfilled only by the provision of adequate health and social measures and

---

[3] Reproduced from *Rio Political Declaration on Social Determinants of Health*, World Health Organization (WHO), Pages 1–7, Copyright 2011. https://www.who.int/publications/m/item/rio-political-declaration-on-social-determinants-of-health. Accessed on August 3, 2022.

that national efforts need to be supported by an enabling international environment.

4. We reaffirm that health inequities within and between countries are politically, socially, and economically unacceptable, as well as unfair and largely avoidable, and that the promotion of health equity is essential to sustainable development and to a better quality of life and well-being for all, which in turn can contribute to peace and security.

5. We reiterate our determination to take action on social determinants of health as collectively agreed by the World Health Assembly and reflected in resolution WHA62.14 ("Reducing health inequities through action on the social determinants of health"), which notes the three overarching recommendations of the Commission on Social Determinants of Health: to improve daily living conditions; to tackle the inequitable distribution of power, money, and resources; and to measure and understand the problem and assess the impact of action.

6. Health inequities arise from the societal conditions in which people are born, grow, live, work, and age, referred to as social determinants of health. These include early years' experiences, education, economic status, employment and decent work, housing and environment, and effective systems of preventing and treating ill health. We are convinced that action on these determinants, both for vulnerable groups and the entire population, is essential to create inclusive, equitable, economically productive, and healthy societies. Positioning human health and well-being as one of the key features of what constitutes a successful, inclusive, and fair society in the twenty-first century is consistent with our commitment to human rights at national and international levels.

7. Good health requires a universal, comprehensive, equitable, effective, responsive, and accessible quality health system. But it is also dependent on the involvement of and dialogue with other sectors and actors, as their performance has significant health impacts. Collaboration in coordinated and intersectoral policy actions has proven to be effective. Health in All Policies, together with intersectoral cooperation and action, is one promising approach to enhance accountability in other sectors for health, as well as the promotion of health equity and more inclusive and productive societies. As collective goals, good health and well-being for all should be given high priority at local, national, regional, and international levels.

8. We recognize that we need to do more to accelerate progress in addressing the unequal distribution of health resources as well as conditions damaging to health at all levels. Based on the experiences shared at this Conference, we express our political will to make health equity a national, regional, and global goal and to address current challenges, such as eradicating hunger and poverty, ensuring food and nutritional security, access to safe drinking water and sanitation, employment and decent work and social protection, protecting environments, and delivering equitable economic growth, through resolute action on social determinants of health across all sectors and at all levels. We

also acknowledge that by addressing social determinants, we can contribute to the achievement of the Millennium Development Goals.

9. The current global economic and financial crisis urgently requires the adoption of actions to reduce increasing health inequities and prevent worsening of living conditions and the deterioration of universal health care and social protection systems.

10. We acknowledge that action on social determinants of health is called for both within countries and at the global level. We underscore that increasing the ability of global actors, through better global governance, promotion of international cooperation and development, participation in policy-making, and monitoring progress, is essential to contribute to national and local efforts on social determinants of health. Action on social determinants of health should be adapted to the national and sub-national contexts of individual countries and regions to take into account different social, cultural, and economic systems. Evidence from research and experiences in implementing policies on social determinants of health, however, shows common features of successful action. There are five key action areas critical to addressing health inequities: (i) to adopt better governance for health and development; (ii) promote participation in policy-making and implementation; (iii) to further reorient the health sector toward reducing health inequities; (iv) to strengthen global governance and collaboration; and (v) to monitor progress and increase accountability. Action on social determinants of health therefore means that we, the representatives of Governments, will strive individually and collectively to develop and support policies, strategies, programs, and action plans, which address social determinants of health, with the support of the international community, that include:

11. *To adopt* better *governance for health and development.*

11.1. Acknowledging that governance to address social determinants involves transparent and inclusive decision-making processes that give voice to all groups and sectors involved and develop policies that perform effectively and reach clear and measurable outcomes, build accountability, and, most crucially, are fair in both policy development processes and results.

11.2. We pledge to:

  (i) Work across different sectors and levels of government, including through, as appropriate, national development strategies, taking into account their contribution to health and health equity and recognizing the leading role of health ministries for advocacy in this regard.

  (ii) Develop policies that are inclusive and take account of the needs of the entire population with specific attention to vulnerable groups and high-risk areas.

  (iii) Support comprehensive programs of research and surveys to inform policy and action.

  (iv) Promote awareness, consideration, and increased accountability of policy-makers for impacts of all policies on health.

   (v) Develop approaches, including effective partnerships, to engage other sectors in order to identify individual and joint roles for improvements in health and reduction of health inequities.

 (vi) Support all sectors in the development of tools and capacities to address social determinants of health at national and international levels.

 (vii) Foster collaboration with the private sector, safeguarding against conflict of interests, to contribute to achieving health through policies and actions on social determinants of health.

(viii) Implement resolution WHA62.14, which takes note of the recommendations of the final report of the Commission on Social Determinants of Health.

 (ix) Strengthen occupational health safety and health protection and their oversight and encourage the public and private sectors to offer healthy working conditions so as to contribute to promoting health for all.

 (x) Promote and strengthen universal access to social services and social protection floors.

 (xi) Give special attention to gender-related aspects as well as early child development in public policies and social and health services.

 (xii) Promote access to affordable, safe, efficacious, and quality medicines, including through the full implementation of the WHO Global Strategy and Plan of Action on Public Health, Innovation and Intellectual Property.

(xiii) Strengthen international cooperation with a view to promoting health equity in all countries through facilitating transfer on mutually agreed terms of expertise, technologies, and scientific data in the field of social determinants of health, as well as exchange of good practices for managing intersectoral policy development.

12. *To promote participation in policy-making and implementation.*

12.1. Acknowledging the importance of participatory processes in policy-making and implementation for effective governance to act on social determinants of health.

12.2. We pledge to:

   (i) Promote and enhance inclusive and transparent decision-making, implementation, and accountability for health and health governance at all levels, including through enhancing access to information, access to justice, and public participation.

 (ii) Empower the role of communities and strengthen civil society contribution to policy-making and implementation by adopting measures to enable their effective participation for the public interest in decision-making.

 (iii) Promote inclusive and transparent governance approaches, which engage early with affected sectors at all levels of governments, as well as support social participation and involve civil society and the private sector, safeguarding against conflict of interests.

(iv) Consider the particular social determinants resulting in persistent health inequities for Indigenous people, in the spirit of the United Nations Declaration on the Rights of Indigenous Peoples, and their specific needs and promote meaningful collaboration with them in the development and delivery of related policies and programs.

(v) Consider the contributions and capacities of civil society to take action in advocacy, social mobilization, and implementation on social determinants of health.

(vi) Promote health equity in all countries particularly through the exchange of good practices regarding increased participation in policy development and implementation.

(vii) Promote the full and effective participation of developed and developing countries in the formulation and implementation of policies and measures to address social determinants of health at the international level.

13. *To further reorient the health sector toward reducing health inequities.*

13.1. Acknowledging that accessibility, availability, acceptability, affordability, and quality of health care and public health services are essential to the enjoyment of the highest attainable standard of health, one of the fundamental rights of every human being, and that the health sector should firmly act to reduce health inequities.

13.2. We pledge to:

(i) Maintain and develop effective public health policies which address the social, economic, environmental, and behavioral determinants of health with a particular focus on reducing health inequities.

(ii) Strengthen health systems toward the provision of equitable universal coverage and promote access to high quality, promotive, preventive, curative, and rehabilitative health services throughout the life cycle, with a particular focus on comprehensive and integrated primary health care.

(iii) Build, strengthen, and maintain public health capacity, including capacity for intersectoral action, on social determinants of health.

(iv) Build, strengthen, and maintain health financing and risk pooling systems that prevent people from becoming impoverished when they seek medical treatment.

(v) Promote mechanisms for supporting and strengthening community initiatives for health financing and risk pooling systems.

(vi) Promote changes within the health sector, as appropriate, to provide the capacities and tools to act to reduce health inequities including through collaborative action.

(vii) Integrate equity, as a priority within health systems, as well as in the design and delivery of health services and public health programs.

(viii) Reach out and work across and within all levels and sectors of government by promoting mechanisms for dialogue, problem-solving, and health impact assessment with an equity focus to identify and promote policies, programs, practices, and legislative measures that may be instrumental for the goal pursued by this Political Declaration and to adapt or reform those harmful to health and health equity.

(ix) Exchange good practices and successful experiences with regard to policies, strategies, and measures to further reorient the health sector toward reducing health inequities.

14. *To strengthen global governance and collaboration.*

14.1. Acknowledging the importance of international cooperation and solidarity for the equitable benefit of all people and the important role the multilateral organizations have in articulating norms and guidelines and identifying good practices for supporting actions on social determinants, and in facilitating access to financial resources and technical cooperation, as well as in reviewing and, where appropriate, strategically modifying policies and practices that have a negative impact on people's health and well-being.

14.2. We pledge to:

(i) Adopt coherent policy approaches that are based on the right to the enjoyment of the highest attainable standard of health, taking into account the right to development as referred to, inter alia, by the 1993 Vienna Declaration and Programme of Action, that will strengthen the focus on social determinants of health, toward achieving the Millennium Development Goals.

(ii) Support social protection floors as defined by countries to address their specific needs and the ongoing work on social protection within the United Nations system, including the work of the International Labour Organization.

(iii) Support national governments, international organizations, nongovernmental entities, and others to tackle social determinants of health as well as to strive to ensure that efforts to advance international development goals and objectives to improve health equity are mutually supportive.

(iv) Accelerate the implementation by the State Parties of the WHO Framework Convention on Tobacco Control (FCTC), recognizing the full range of measures including measures to reduce consumption and availability, and encourage countries that have not yet done so to consider acceding to the FCTC as we recognize that substantially reducing tobacco consumption is an important contribution to addressing social determinants of health and vice versa.

(v) Take forward the actions set out in the political declaration of the United Nations General Assembly High-Level Meeting on the Prevention and Control Noncommunicable Diseases at local, national, and international levels—ensuring a focus on reducing health inequities.

(vi) Support the leading role of the World Health Organization in global health governance, and in promoting alignment in policies, plans, and activities on social determinants of health with its partner United Nations agencies, development banks, and other key international organizations, including in joint advocacy, and in facilitating access to the provision of financial and technical assistance to countries and regions.

(vii) Support the efforts of governments to promote capacity and establish incentives to create a sustainable workforce in health and in other fields, especially in areas of greatest need.

(viii) Build capacity of national governments to address social determinants of health by facilitating expertise and access to resources through appropriate United Nations agencies' support, particularly the World Health Organization.

(ix) Foster North-South and South-South cooperation in showcasing initiatives, building capacity, and facilitating the transfer of technology on mutually agreed terms for integrated action on health inequities, in line with national priorities and needs, including on health services and pharmaceutical production, as appropriate.

15. *To monitor progress and increase accountability.*

15.1. Acknowledging that monitoring of trends in health inequities and of impacts of actions to tackle them is critical to achieving meaningful progress, that information systems should facilitate the establishment of relationships between health outcomes and social stratification variables, and that accountability mechanisms to guide policy-making in all sectors are essential, taking into account different national contexts.

15.2. We pledge to:

(i) Establish, strengthen, and maintain monitoring systems that provide disaggregated data to assess inequities in health outcomes as well as in allocations and use of resources.

(ii) Develop and implement robust, evidence-based, reliable measures of societal well-being, building where possible on existing indicators, standards, and programs and across the social gradient that go beyond economic growth.

(iii) Promote research on the relationships between social determinants and health equity outcomes with a particular focus on evaluation of effectiveness of interventions.

(iv) Systematically share relevant evidence and trends among different sectors to inform policy and action.

(v) Improve access to the results of monitoring and research for all sectors in society.

(vi) Assess the impacts of policies on health and other societal goals, and take these into account in policy-making.

(vii) Use intersectoral mechanisms such as a Health in All Policies approach for addressing inequities and social determinants of health; enhance access to justice and ensure accountability, which can be followed up.

(viii) Support the leading role of the World Health Organization in its collaboration with other United Nations agencies in strengthening the monitoring of progress in the field of social determinants of health and in providing guidance and support to Member States in implementing a Health in All Policies approach to tackling inequities in health.

(ix) Support the World Health Organization on the follow-up to the recommendations of the Commission on Information and Accountability for Women's and Children's Health.

(x) Promote appropriate monitoring systems that take into consideration the role of all relevant stakeholders including civil society, nongovernmental organizations, as well as the private sector, with appropriate safeguard against conflict of interests, in the monitoring and evaluation process.

(xi) Promote health equity in and among countries, monitoring progress at the international level and increasing collective accountability in the field of social determinants of health, particularly through the exchange of good practices in this field.

(xii) Improve universal access to and use of inclusive information technologies and innovation in key social determinants of health.

16. *Call for global action.*

16.1. We, Heads of Government, Ministers, and government representatives, solemnly reaffirm our resolve to take action on social determinants of health to create vibrant, inclusive, equitable, economically productive, and healthy societies and to overcome national, regional, and global challenges to sustainable development. We offer our solid support for these common objectives and our determination to achieve them.

16.2. We call upon the World Health Organization, United Nations agencies, and other international organizations to advocate for, coordinate, and collaborate with us in the implementation of these actions. We recognize that global action on social determinants will need increased capacity and knowledge within the World Health Organization and other multilateral organizations for the development and sharing of norms, standards, and good practices. Our common values and responsibilities toward humanity move us to fulfill our pledge to act on social determinants of health. We firmly believe that doing so is not only a moral and a human rights imperative but also indispensable to promote human well-being, peace, prosperity, and sustainable development. We call upon the international community to support developing countries in the implementation of these actions through the exchange of best practices, the provision of technical assistance, and in facilitating access to financial resources, while reaffirming the provisions of the United Nations Millennium Declaration as well as the Monterrey Consensus of the International Conference on Financing for Development.

16.3. We urge those developed countries which have pledged to achieve the target of 0.7% of GNP for official development assistance by 2015, and those developed countries that have not yet done so, to make additional concrete efforts to fulfill their commitments in this regard. We also urge developing countries to build on progress achieved in ensuring that official development assistance is used effectively to help achieve development goals and targets.

16.4. World leaders will soon gather again here in Rio de Janeiro to consider how to meet the challenge of sustainable development laid down 20 years ago. This Political Declaration recognizes the important policies needed to achieve both sustainable development and health equity through acting on social determinants.

16.5. We recommend that the social determinants approach is duly considered in the ongoing reform process of the World Health Organization. We also recommend that the 65th World Health Assembly adopts a resolution endorsing this Political Declaration.

Appendix D: Human Rights and Health (Fact Sheet)[4]

Key Facts

- The WHO Constitution (1946) envisages "…the highest attainable standard of health as a fundamental right of every human being."
- Understanding health as a human right creates a legal obligation on states to ensure access to timely, acceptable, and affordable health care of appropriate quality as well as to providing for the underlying determinants of health, such as safe and potable water, sanitation, food, housing, health-related information and education, and gender equality.
- A States' obligation to support the right to health—including through the allocation of "maximum available resources" to progressively realize this goal—is reviewed through various international human rights mechanisms, such as the Universal Periodic Review, or the Committee on Economic, Social and Cultural Rights. In many cases, the right to health has been adopted into domestic law or Constitutional law.
- A rights-based approach to health requires that health policy and programs must prioritize the needs of those furthest behind first toward greater equity, a principle that has been echoed in the recently adopted 2030 Agenda for Sustainable Development and Universal Health Coverage (1).

---

[4] Reproduced from *Human Rights and Health*, World Health Organization (WHO), Copyright 2017. https://www.who.int/news-room/fact-sheets/detail/human-rights-and-health. Accessed on July 8, 2022.

- The right to health must be enjoyed without discrimination on the grounds of race, age, ethnicity, or any other status. Non-discrimination and equality requires states to take steps to redress any discriminatory law, practice, or policy.
- Another feature of rights-based approaches is meaningful participation. Participation means ensuring that national stakeholders—including non-state actors such as nongovernmental organizations—are meaningfully involved in all phases of programming: assessment, analysis, planning, implementation, monitoring, and evaluation.

"The right to the highest attainable standard of health" implies a clear set of legal obligations on states to ensure appropriate conditions for the enjoyment of health for all people without discrimination.

The right to health is one of a set of internationally agreed human rights standards and is inseparable or "indivisible" from these other rights. This means achieving the right to health is both central to, and dependent upon, the realization of other human rights, to food, housing, work, education, information, and participation.

The right to health, as with other rights, includes both freedoms and entitlements:

- Freedoms include the right to control one's health and body (e.g., sexual and reproductive rights) and to be free from interference (e.g., free from torture and non-consensual medical treatment and experimentation).
- Entitlements include the right to a system of health protection that gives everyone an equal opportunity to enjoy the highest attainable level of health.

Focus on Disadvantaged Populations

Disadvantage and marginalization serve to exclude certain populations in societies from enjoying good health. Three of the world's most fatal communicable diseases—malaria, HIV/AIDS, and tuberculosis—disproportionately affect the world's poorest populations and in many cases are compounded and exacerbated by other inequalities and inequities including gender, age, sexual orientation or gender identity, and migration status. Conversely the burden of noncommunicable diseases—often perceived as affecting high-income countries—is increasing disproportionately among lower-income countries and populations and is largely associated with lifestyle and behavior factors as well as environmental determinants, such as safe housing, water, and sanitation that are inextricably linked to human rights.

A focus on disadvantage also reveals evidence of those who are exposed to greater rates of ill-health and face significant obstacles to accessing quality and affordable health care, including Indigenous populations. While data collection systems are often ill-equipped to capture data on these groups, reports show that these populations have higher mortality and morbidity rates, due to noncommunicable diseases such as cancer, cardiovascular diseases, and chronic respiratory disease. These populations may also be the subject of laws and policies that further compound their marginalization and make it harder for them to access healthcare prevention, treatment, rehabilitation, and care services.

Violations of Human Rights in Health

Violations or lack of attention to human rights can have serious health consequences. Overt or implicit discrimination in the delivery of health services—both within the health workforce and between health workers and service users—acts as a powerful barrier to health services and contributes to poor quality care.

Mental ill-health often leads to a denial of dignity and autonomy, including forced treatment or institutionalization, and disregard of individual legal capacity to make decisions. Paradoxically, mental health is still given inadequate attention in public health, in spite of the high levels of violence, poverty, and social exclusion that contribute to worse mental and physical health outcomes for people with mental health disorders.

Violations of human rights not only contribute to and exacerbate poor health, but for many, including people with disabilities, Indigenous populations, women living with HIV, sex workers, people who use drugs, transgender, and intersex people, the healthcare setting presents a risk of heightened exposure to human rights abuses—including coercive or forced treatment and procedures.

Human Rights-Based Approaches

A human rights-based approach to health provides a set of clear principles for setting and evaluating health policy and service delivery, targeting discriminatory practices and unjust power relations that are at the heart of inequitable health outcomes.

In pursuing a rights-based approach, health policy, strategies, and programs should be designed explicitly to improve the enjoyment of all people to the right to health, with a focus on the furthest behind first. The core principles and standards of a rights-based approach are detailed below.

Core Principles of Human Rights

Accountability

States and other duty-bearers are answerable for the observance of human rights. However, there is also a growing movement recognizing the importance of other non-state actors such as businesses in the respect and protection of human rights (2).

Equality and Non-discrimination

The principle of non-discrimination seeks "…to guarantee that human rights are exercised without discrimination of any kind based on race, colour, sex, language, religion, political, or other opinion, national or social origin, property, birth or other status such as disability, age, marital and family status, sexual orientation and gender identity, health status, place of residence, economic and social situation."

Any discrimination, for example, in access to health care, as well as in means and entitlements for achieving this access, is prohibited on the basis of race, color, sex, language, religion, political or other opinion, national or social origin, property, birth, physical or mental disability, health status (including HIV/AIDS), sexual orientation, and civil, political, social, or other status, which has the intention or effect of impairing the equal enjoyment or exercise of the right to health.

The principle of non-discrimination and equality requires the WHO to address discrimination in guidance, policies, and practices, such as relating to the distribution and provision of resources and health services. Non-discrimination and equality are key measures required to address the social determinants affecting the enjoyment of the right to health. Functioning national health information systems and availability of disaggregated data are essential to be able to identify the most vulnerable groups and diverse needs.

Participation

Participation requires ensuring that all concerned stakeholders including non-state actors have ownership and control over development processes in all phases of the programming cycle: assessment, analysis, planning, implementation, monitoring, and evaluation. Participation goes well beyond consultation or a technical addition to project design; it should include explicit strategies to empower citizens, especially the most marginalized, so that their expectations are recognized by the State.

Participation is important to accountability as it provides "…checks and balances which do not allow unitary leadership to exercise power in an arbitrary manner."

Universal, Indivisible, and Interdependent

Human rights are universal and inalienable. They apply equally, to all people, everywhere, without distinction. Human rights standards—to food, health, education, and be free from torture, inhuman, or degrading treatment—are also interrelated. The improvement of one right facilitates advancement of the others. Likewise, the deprivation of one right adversely affects the others.

Core Elements of a Right to Health

Progressive Realization Using Maximum Available Resources

No matter what level of resources they have at their disposal, progressive realization requires that governments take immediate steps within their means toward the fulfillment of these rights. Regardless of resource capacity, the elimination of discrimination and improvements in the legal and juridical systems must be acted upon with immediate effect.

Non-retrogression

States should not allow the existing protection of economic, social, and cultural rights to deteriorate unless there are strong justifications for a retrogressive measure. For example, introducing school fees in secondary education which had formerly been free of charge would constitute a deliberate retrogressive measure. To justify it, a State would have to demonstrate that it adopted the measure only after carefully considering all the options, assessing the impact and fully using its maximum available resources.

Core Components of the Right to Health

The right to health (Article 12) was defined in General Comment 14 of the Committee on Economic, Social and Cultural Rights—a committee of Independent Experts, responsible for overseeing adherence to the Covenant (4). The right includes the following core components:

Availability

Refers to the need for a sufficient quantity of functioning public health and healthcare facilities, goods, and services, as well as programs for all. Availability can be measured through the analysis of disaggregated data to different and multiple stratifiers including by age, sex, location, and socioeconomic status and qualitative surveys to understand coverage gaps and health workforce coverage

Accessibility

Requires that health facilities, goods, and services must be accessible to everyone. Accessibility has four overlapping dimensions:

- Non-discrimination.
- Physical accessibility.
- Economical accessibility (affordability).
- Information accessibility.

Assessing accessibility may require analysis of barriers—physical financial or otherwise—that exist, and how they may affect the most vulnerable, and call for the establishment or application of clear norms and standards in both law and policy to address these barriers, as well as robust monitoring systems of health-related information and whether this information is reaching all populations.

Acceptability

Relates to respect for medical ethics, culturally appropriate, and sensitivity to gender. Acceptability requires that health facilities, goods, services, and programs are people-centered and cater for the specific needs of diverse population groups and in accordance with international standards of medical ethics for confidentiality and informed consent.

Quality

Facilities, goods, and services must be scientifically and medically approved. Quality is a key component of Universal Health Coverage and includes the experience as well as the perception of health care. Quality health services should be:

- Safe—avoiding injuries to people for whom the care is intended.
- Effective—providing evidence-based healthcare services to those who need them.
- People-centered—providing care that responds to individual preferences, needs, and values.
- Timely—reducing waiting times and sometimes harmful delays.
- Equitable—providing care that does not vary in quality on account of gender, ethnicity, geographic location, and socioeconomic status.
- Integrated—providing care that makes available the full range of health services throughout the life course.
- Efficient—maximizing the benefit of available resources and avoiding waste.

WHO Response

The WHO has made a commitment to mainstream human rights into healthcare programs and policies on national and regional levels by looking at underlying determinants of health as part of a comprehensive approach to health and human rights.

In addition, the WHO has been actively strengthening its role in providing technical, intellectual, and political leadership on the right to health including:

- Strengthening the capacity of the WHO and its Member States to integrate a human rights-based approach to health.
- Advancing the right to health in international law and international development processes.
- Advocating for health-related human rights, including the right to health.

Addressing the needs and rights of individuals at different stages across the life course requires taking a comprehensive approach within the broader context of promoting human rights, gender equality, and equity.

As such, the WHO promotes a concise and unifying framework that builds on existing approaches in gender, equity, and human rights to generate more accurate and robust solutions to health inequities. The integrated nature of the framework is an opportunity to build on foundational strengths and complementarities between these approaches to create a cohesive and efficient approach to promote health and well-being for all.

1. Transforming our World: The 2030 Agenda for Sustainable Development.
   UN General Assembly. 2015. 21 October. UN Doc. A/RES/70/1.
2. General comment No. 20: Non-discrimination in economic, social and cultural rights.
   Committee on Economic, Social and Cultural Rights. 2009.
3. Guiding principles for business and human rights, Implementing the United Nations "Protect, Respect and Remedy" Framework.
   Office of the high Commissioner for Human Rights, Geneva, 2011.
4. CESCR General Comment No. 14: The Right to the Highest Attainable Standard of Health
   (Art. 12). CESCR (Committee on Economic, Social, and Cultural Rights). 2000.). 11 August. Doc. E/C.12/2000/4.

References

Amadeo, K. (2021). *The impact of WWII*. Retrieved March 6, 2022, from https://www.thebalance.com/world-war-ii-economic-impact-4570917

Backman, G., Hunt, P., Khosla, R., Jaramillo-Strouss, C., Mekuria Fikre, B., Rumble, C., Pevalin, D., Acurio Páez, D., Armijos Pineda, M., Frisancho, A., Tarco, D., Motlagh, M., Farcasanu, D., & Vladescu, C. (2008). Health systems and the right to health: An assessment of 194 countries. *Lancet, 372*, 2047–2085. https://doi.org/10.1016/S0140-6736(08)61781-X

Blix, B., Hamran, T., & Normann, H. (2012). Indigenous life stories as narratives of health and resistance: A dialogical narrative analysis. *CJNR, 44*(2), 64–85.

Browne, A. (2000). The potential contributions of critical social theory to nursing science. *Canadian Journal of Nursing, 32*(2), 35–55.

Bunker, S. (2010). A focus on human flourishing. *Nursing Science Quarterly, 23*(4), 290–295. https://doi.org/10.1177/0894318410380258

Burnett, C., Swanberg, M., Hudson, A., & Schminkey, D. (2018). Structural justice: A critical feminist framework exploring the intersection between justice, equity and structural reconciliation. *Journal of Health Disparities Research and Practice, 11*(4), 52–68.

Card, A. (2019). Flourishing as a definition of health. *JAMA, 322*(10), 981. https://doi.org/10.1001/jama.2019.10343

Cowling, W. R., Chinn, P. L., & Hagedorn, S. (2000, April 30). *A nursing manifesto: A call to conscience and action.* Retrieved May 16, 2021, from http://www.nursemanifest.com/manifesto_num.htm

Davis, O. (2013, Summer). Barbershop cuisine: African American foodways and narratives of health in the black barbershop. *International Journal of Men's Health, 12*(2), 138–149. https://doi.org/10.3149/jmh.1202.138.19

Hatala, A., Dejardins, M., & Bombay, A. (2016). Reframing narratives of aboriginal health inequity: Exploring cree elder resilience and well-being in contexts of historical trauma. *Qualitative Health Research, 26*(14), 1911–1927. https://doi.org/10.1177/1049732315609569

Huber, M., Knottnerus, J., Green, L., der Horstead, H., Jadad, A., Kromhout, D., Leonard, B., Lorig, K., Loureiro, M., van der Meer, J., Schnabel, P., Smith, R., Weelhead, C., & Smid, H. (2011). How should we define health? *BMJ, 343*, d4163. https://doi.org/10.1136/bmj.d4163

Jakarta Declaration on health promotion into the 21st century. (1998). Rev Panam Salud Publica/*Pan American Journal of Public Health*, *3*(1). Retrieved March 27, 2021, from https://scielosp.org/pdf/rpsp/1998.v3n1/58-61/en

Kagan, P., Smith, M., Cowling, W., & Chin, P. (2010). A nursing manifesto: An emancipatory call for knowledge development, conscience, and praxis. *Nursing Philosophy, 11*, 67–84. https://doi.org/10.1111/j.1466-769X.2009.00422.x

Misselbrook, D. (2014). W is for Well-being and the WHO definition of health, *British Journal of General Practice*, *64*(628), 582. https://doi.org/10.3399/bjgp14X682381. Retrieved March 6, 2021, from https://bjgp.org/content/bjgp/64/628/582.full.pdf.

The World Health Organization. (2017). *Health as a human rights fact sheet.* Retrieved July 8, 2022, from https://www.who.int/news-room/fact-sheets/detail/human-rights-and-health

Toronto Declaration on Equity in Health. (2002). *Rev Panam Salud Publica/Pan Am J Public Health*, *12*(6). Retrieved April 3, 2021, from https://www.scielosp.org/pdf/rpsp/2002.v12n6/465-467/en

United Nations General Assembly. (2012). *The future we want.* Resolution A/RES/66/288, Adopted July 27, 2021. Retrieved April 10, from https://sustainabledevelopment.un.org/futurewewant.html

Vanderweele, T. (2017, August 1). On the promotion of human flourishing. *Proceedings of the National Academy of Sciences of the United States of America*, *114*(31). Retrieved from: www.pnas.org/cgi/doi/10.1073/pnas.1702996114

Wesp, L., Scheer, V., Ruiz, A., Walker, K., Weitzel, J., Shaw, L., Kako, P., & Mkandawire-Valhmu, L., (2018, October/December). An emancipatory approach to cultural competency. *Advances in Nursing Science, 41*(4), 316–326. https://doi.org/10.1097/ANS.0000000000000230.

Williams, C., & Mikola, M. (2018). From multiculturalism to superdiversity? Narratives of health and wellbeing in an urban neighborhood, social work & policy studies. *Social Justice, Practice and Theory, 1*(1).

Williamson, & Carr. (2009, March). Health as a resource for everyday life: Advancing the conceptualization. *Critical Public Health, 19*(1), 107–122.

World Health Organization. (1946). *WHO: Official records of the WHO meeting.* Retrieved March 1, 2022, from https://apps.who.int/iris/bitstream/handle/10665/85573/Official_record2_eng.pdf?sequence=1&isAllowed=y

World Health Organization. (1986). *The Ottawa charter.* Retrieved March 1, 2022, from https://www.who.int/teams/health-promotion/enhanced-wellbeing/first-global-conference

World Health Organization. (1997). *The WHO Jakarta declaration on leading health promotion into the 20th century.* Retrieved March 27, 2021, from https://www.who.int/healthpromotion/conferences/previous/jakarta/declaration/en/

World Health Organization. (2011). *World conference on the social the social determinants of health: Rio.* Retrieved April 3, 2021, from https://www.who.int/publications/m/item/rio-political-declaration-on-social-determinants-of-health

Chapter 2
Contextualizing and Situating Race and Health in the United States

In the United States and arguably globally, we face ever-increasing health disparities and widening inequity gaps especially among Black, Brown, Asian, Latinx, and Indigenous peoples. These populations have historically been subjugated, intentionally excluded, and marginalized, causing generational devastation in their social, economic, and health outcomes. Routinely, racialized populations disproportionately suffer from higher rates of several health-related (health disparities, chronic disease, morbidity, and mortality) and social consequences (such as poverty, limited access to opportunity and services, decreased social mobility, and racism) that diminish life expectancy and quality of life. Direct and indirect impacts of cumulative and intersecting exposure to these consequences produce chronic challenges that are further exacerbated by structures (institutions, policies, practices, and institutional agents), the inequitable distribution of power and privilege, and importantly the history of race and health in this country.

2.1 History of Race and Health in the United States

The healthcare profession has not been insulated from racist practices and beliefs. In fact, there is a long-standing history of medical abuses rooted in racism (segregation, eugenics, sterilization, experimentation, withholding treatment/treatment without consent, and exclusion) used by the healthcare system and professionals. Racist ideologies (false narratives about race, tolerance to conditions, centering whiteness) have been embedded in the education of healthcare providers for decades, while representation of the diverse composition of healthcare providers wanes, further negatively affecting the lives of the most marginalized.

In the aftermath of many successive racially motivated murders that peaked in the summer of 2020, several professional healthcare organizations were compelled by public and professional outcry to redress their own long-known racist history and practices, out loud. This meant acknowledging the historical role that those and institutions entrusted to provide care have played in racism and then starting to reconcile this dark history with identifying and implementing better principles and practices moving forward.

C. Burnett, *Justice in Health*, https://doi.org/10.1007/978-3-031-18504-5_2

2.1.1 Medical Abuses of Black Bodies

Black people have been the subject of medical abuses in the form of research, medical procedures, and the experimentation that began during slavery. African Americans, who were forcefully removed from Africa and brought to the United States for slavery, used traditional healing practices and remedies for treatment. When arriving in the United States, they were subjected to physical examination and inspections by physicians who determined their suitability to bear the brutality they were about to endure. These physicians signed "certificates of soundness" which were used to estimate the market value of the slaves and became a key "professional competencies needed by southern doctors" to help insurance companies and slave owners protect their asset (Owens & Fett, 2019, p. 1432). These medical abuses persisted, and the racialized pursuit of science continued. Race was intentionally crafted as a construct used to justify difference in human beings by categorizing human traits with corresponding rankings of superior to inferior. Moreover, the emergence of the scientific narrative of Black inferiority and difference based on a social construction of race fueled justification for these injustices and were legitimized by physicians and natural scientists (Byrd & Clayton, 2001). Witzig (1996) and others (Nieblas-Bedolla et al., 2020; Wolf et al., 2020) confirm that the concept of race is pathologically unfounded and unscientific, and the terms destructiveness have "fueled racist and eugenic movements with allegedly scientific claims of racial superiority and inferiority" (Witzig, 1996, p. 676). Even recently the AMA report (2021) identified that "race is a socially constructed way of grouping people based on skin color and other apparent physical differences. It has been defined by an arbitrarily organized combination of physical traits, geographic ancestry, language, religion and variety of cultural features (p. 13)."

With the help and encouragement of the unsubstantiated medical science of race as a biological difference, Blacks were perceived and labeled inferior to Whites. This allowed Blacks to be viewed as less human and created the moral cover to dehumanize them in the most egregious ways and centered them as subjects of fodder for curiosity, experimentation, and outright exploitation.

There was the painful experimentation of Black women in the development of gynecological procedures that produced the cure for vesicovaginal fistula, perfecting of the cesarean section and the ovariotomy (Owens & Fett, 2019; Dula, 1994, Savitt, 1982). Ironically while purporting diminished intellect of Black people, Black women's nursing knowledge was heavily relied upon to assist these same physicians in conducting the experimental gynecological surgeries. A recent 2022 report by the National Commission on Racism in Nursing captures this juxtaposition in their findings:

> …But even as white physicians assumed that enslaved women were intellectually inferior, using their perceived intellectual and biological differences as justification for their enslavement and for the violence enacted upon them in the name of medical experimentation, they nevertheless relied on enslaved women to work as nurses and surgical assistants—work which required high levels of skill and in which intelligence and judgment were valued. Collectively, this scholarship on the nursing work of enslaved women highlights, as

R.J. Knight recently summed up, that the work of enslaved nurses "encompassed exploitation and power as much as intimacy and care, forced labor as well as free, and has served
both communities and regimes (Tobbell & D'Antonio, 2022, p. 12).

Grave robbing of Black people to exploit their cadavers involved medical schools
purchasing or stealing these bodies for dissection, training, and education of their
students (Dula, 1994). African Americans were particularly susceptible to this
widespread indignation given their marginalized social status that affected where
and how they were buried and the overall devaluation for their personhood (Highet,
2005). Given the pervasive sentiment of white superiority, the desecration of Black
corpses to pursue medical advancement was accepted:

The issue of grave robbing once out of sight seems to have been safely out of mind for upper
class citizens, despite the terrorizing grip it continued to hold over the lower classes. The
rampant social discrimination embraced by the medical community of this era was wrapped
up by many layers of hypocrisy. Conveniently enough, despite the pretense that Caucasian
and African American bodies were inherently different enough to warrant a separate medical science and practice for each group, it was nevertheless accepted that the information
gained through dissecting African American cadavers could make valuable contributions to
so-called "white" medicine (Savitt 1982: 332). It was further popularly proposed that so
long as only the bodies of African Americans and the indigent—who presumably leached
resources from society—were used for dissection, nobody should object to this practice
since it offered these groups an opportunity to repay their "debt" to society (Highet, 2005,
pp. 421–422).

Demand for medical schools that could offer the dissecting experience to teaching
anatomy as a reflection of the quality and standard of their medical education fueled
the need for an increasing supply of cadavers. Medical school reputations were built
and sustained on their ability to obtain and supply human specimens for teaching
purposes, and these specimens were predominantly Black and poor. Savitt (1982)
recounts the fierce competition for students by southern medical school whereby
these institutions publicized "the positive aspects of its programs": "One of the
major requisites of any school were an abundant supply of clinical material-living
patients for medical and surgical demonstrations as well as cadavers for anatomical
dissections and pathological examinations" (Savitt, 1982, p. 333). This and other
horrendous behaviors by those whose most sacred professional oath is to do no
harm have caused irreparable damage to the trust between patient and healthcare
professionals and the overall medical establishment. These are some of the many
historical seeds that contribute to the disparities and mistrust of medicine.

Other gross violations of sacred relationship with the public involve the involuntary, deceptive, and/or coercive sterilization of individuals well into the early 1970s
through government sponsorship (Dula, 1994; Borrero et al., 2012; Reilly, 2015).
Early eugenics beliefs about the need to protect the human gene pool were embraced
by US biologist Charles Davenport and physician Dr. Harvey Sharp spurring US
sterilization laws targeting those deemed to be "unfit" such as the incarcerated,
institutionalized, and those with mental disabilities (Reilly, 1987, 2015). These
early laws evolved overtime to include the poor, Black, Native American, and immigrant women. In 1948, it was reported that "welfare workers in North Carolina
provided sterilization services to more than 150 young, mostly black women who

were neither mentally deficient nor institutionalized" (Reilly, 2015, p. 359). These sterilizations continued well into the 1960s and 1970s with documented cases of deceptive sterilizations of Mexican immigrant women and involuntary sterilization of Black and Native American women (Reilly, 2015).

Without the endorsement and active involvement of the medicalization of race over centuries, the depth and breadth of the brutalization of Black bodies could not have been sustained, let alone encouraged. Abuses occurred at many access points internal and external to the formal system of care and were encountered more globally within the scientific community and predominantly in the name of advancement of science.

Research abuses have been widely documented for centuries. Thomas Jefferson allowed the unconsented inoculation of 200 of his slaves to test the smallpox vaccine to ensure it was safe for whites (Dula, 1994). Notably the Tuskegee Study (1932–1972) intentionally withheld education and treatment for syphilis from 399 Black men to study the progression of the disease (Kennedy et al., 2007). Also appalling was this experiment's use of trust to violate poor rural Black populations through needs-based incentives (food, transportation), the involvement of government, and those of respected community agencies and the hiring of a Black nurse for the 40-year duration (Thomas & Quinn, 1991). This study is often referred to as the source of mistrust by African Americans and, however, is one part of the long history of medical abuses that have contributed to those sentiments. The extent of the deception of the Tuskegee experiment encompassed the deliberate withholding of information and worse treatment leading to mortality and morbidity. People's lives were shortened; families and children were intentionally exposed to a preventable debilitating disease. Choice was taken from them and those who were unwitting victims of the study. The study was predatory in seeking out of the most vulnerable and taking the fullest advantage of that vulnerability. Trusted community resource agencies were integrated into the exploitation and a community member from the community and representing a profession that is esteemed as trustworthy played key roles sustaining the engagement of deceived individuals.

2.1.2   Segregation in Health Care

In many parts of the United States, segregation existed in healthcare settings, hospital units, and even within the education of healthcare providers. Education has been and continues to be a highly segregated space divided along race and class. The period of time during the emergence of a formalized education system for physician and nursing training was also very segregated. As Byrd and Clayton (2001) confirm, "the data suggest the foundations of the American health delivery system was built on a class stratified, racially segregated, and discriminatory basis" (p. 125). In fact, the Hill-Burton Act of 1946 funded the US state hospital systems in a federal state partnership that entailed the separate but equal concession requested by Southern states which allowed for segregated care along racial lines (Largent, 2018).

Segregation impacted the training and practicing privileges of Black healthcare providers and where Black people could receive care, which could be a wing, segregated unit, or at a limited handful of Black hospitals, if there was space (Cornely, 1956; Largent, 2018; Education and employment opportunities for Black healthcare professionals were limited and professional association affiliation were outright denied in the South (Cornely, 1956). The impact of this segregation is confounded by many layers of segregation within the community (housing); neighborhoods have played a critical role in the many disparities that we continue to see in diverse populations.

Arnett et al. (2016) reflect that "although segregation of health care was made illegal by the Civil Rights Act of 1964 and Medicare in 1965, de facto segregation of healthcare systems persists as a natural extension of residential segregation (p. 458)." These same authors propose a framework for understanding the impact that segregation has on health disparities in the Black community by its creation of "disparate exposures to healthcare access and quality between African American and white communities (Arnett et al., 2016, p. 458)."

This health disparity has been further reified by race-based diagnostics created by using race in the development of clinical diagnosis. Measures of pulmonary function which "adjusts results of spirometry tests based on the assumption that black people have naturally lower lung function than whites" can potentially cause "serious problems to be missed" (Hostetter & Klein, 2021, p. 10). The race correcting measure of the estimated glomerular rate (estimator of kidney function) significantly impacts diagnosis and severity of kidney disease negatively affecting Black patients' health outcomes (Hostetter & Klein, 2021, p. 11). Race, as the root for falsely constructing a narrative of difference, is the culprit in many of the health disparities that we witness today and helps deepen our understanding as to why they continue.

Segregation of hospitals and access to professional affiliation and education has limited the opportunity of Black healthcare providers' entry and flourishing in the healthcare field, causing underrepresentation that still persists. Jones and Saines (2019) speak to the historical segregation of nurses through their exclusion to various training programs, associations (including the American Nurses Association and the American Red Cross), and service in the US Military Medical Corps. Specifically they identify:

> that few programs admitted black nurses and "black communities responded to such exclusion by pooling resources to establish Black hospitals and hospital based nurse training programs" (Jones & Saines, 2019, p. 878) and that "…associations in 16 states and the District of Columbia excluded Black nurses, effectively barring them from membership on the American Nurses Association (Jones & Saines, 2019, p. 878)

Meanwhile the American Medical Association (AMA) steadfastly upheld discriminatory practices that also include segregated training and exclusionary practices. Their recent report entitled "Organizational Strategic Plan to Embed Racial Justice and Advance Equity 2021–2023," identified that "exclusion from AMA membership created direct barriers to specialty training and professional development for

Black physicians, directly harming minority communities who suffered from a dearth of access to qualified physicians. For example, "in 1993, there were 25,000 subspecialty trained physicians in the United States and only 2 of them were Black" (American Medical Association, 2021, p. 27).

These practices not only created segregation, but also segregated access to opportunity and both professional and social mobility. The effects of limited access to the field of health care still play out today in the underrepresentation of minorities in all health professions, academia, and research, to name a few. In turn this underrepresentation affects patient care, types of research, and education curriculum. It has been reported by Hostetter and Klein (2021) that "the percentage of black physicians has not increased in 80 years" and that with closure of 5 of the 7 nations Black medical colleges there is now "30,000–36,000 fewer black physicians" (p. 21) This is alarming for obvious reasons but also because patients are more likely to visit and trust healthcare providers who look like them.

2.1.3   Underrepresentation of Providers of Color

The representation of minoritized and racialized healthcare providers in relation to the general population is unmatched. While African Americans, Latinos, Alaskan Natives, and American Indians account for 33% of the general population, they represent less than 12% of US physicians (Kendrick et al., 2020, 2021). According to Saizan et al. (2021), it is estimated that "by 2060, more than 50% of Americans will identify as a race other than white" (Rivera-Nieves & Abreu, 2013). Yet less than 12% of physicians in 2018 were underrepresented in medicine (UIM) with African Americans, who comprise 13% of the general population, accounting for only 5% of US physicians (Association of American Medical Colleges, 2018). These numbers are even more striking within healthcare leadership, with 98% of healthcare organization leaders being White (Castillo & Guo, 2011). Racial and ethnic minorities are underrepresented in other sectors of medicine, making up roughly "19.2% and 8% of registered nurses and PhD investigators", respectively (American Association of Colleges of Nursing, 2021; Blanchard et al., 2021) (p. 1)." These statistics emphasize the urgent need to address real gaps in patient/provider racial concordance and the systematic homogeneity in the medical workforce, which has been documented to negatively impact health outcomes, particularly among those from underserved backgrounds as well as racial and ethnic minorities.

There are many reasons why having providers that reflect the populations they serve are important and necessary; first and foremost its effectiveness in helping to improve health outcomes. According to Goode and Landefeld (2018) "Considerable evidence has now been published that increasing the number of healthcare providers from diverse backgrounds, including those from underrepresented racial and ethnic groups, rural communities, and low socioeconomic status (SES), is a vital step in tackling both the projected primary-care physician shortage and healthcare disparities, as well as providing more patient-centered and patient-concordant care" (p. 75). Evidence supports that having more diverse healthcare providers decreases health disparities and improves quality of care and access to care (Clayborne et al., 2021). Racial concordance between provider and patient increases patient engagement and rating of their provider. Exposure to diverse providers not only enhances student training experiences, but students from diverse backgrounds are also more likely to serve in underserved areas (Anachebe, 2021; Clayborne et al., 2021; Wilta et al., 2003).

Beyond provider and patient concordance, diverse providers and scientists are paramount to shaping the future of scientific inquiry. Diverse representation by both ethnicity and gender in sciences and engineering has not significantly improved even though advances in science and technology have steadily increased exponentially.

Access to the brilliance of all minds is what will catalyze new and increasingly critical discoveries and not simply the contributions of only a few. Harnessing the talents and experiences from diverse peoples introduces innovation of ideas that are highly useful to advance important areas of scientific. It also makes economic sense. According to Varma (2018), improving gender and ethnic diversity in the US technology workforce represents a massive economic opportunity, one that could create $470–579 billion in value for the technology company and could add 1.2–1.6% to national gross domestic product. In other words, having women and minorities in technology companies would be good for the business.

Research institutions and funders have taken notice fueling requests for proposals in support of diverse scholars. The Freeman Hrabowski Scholars have recently pledged 1.5 billion dollars toward recruiting biomedical researchers to advance diversity, equity, and inclusion. The focus is on mentorship of trainees from diverse racial and ethnic backgrounds that are underrepresented in science (Howard Hughes Medical Center, 2022). The National Institutes of Health provides diversity supplements (https://grants.nih.gov/grants/guide/contacts/Diversity-Supp_contacts.html) to their awards to encourage inclusion of diverse research scientists and facilitate an opportunity to build a sustainable research career pathway. These efforts to increase diversity of investigators and practitioners is a strategic effort to mitigate health disparities by increasing those researchers and practitioner most likely to pursuit scientific solutions to inequity and devote their practice to populations suffering from health disparities.

2.2 Trajectory of Disparities

Recent US disparities data (Ndugga & Atria, 2021) show that Blacks still fare far worse than their counterparts and Whites across many health status measures such as infant mortality rates, HIV, prevalence of chronic conditions, overall physical and mental health status, most likely to be uninsured, and suffering the highest mortality rates. This report also identified lower health status among the poor and in some cases reported health challenges in LGBTQIA+ populations. COVID-19 only confirmed the disproportionate burden of death and illness that at-risk populations such as Blacks, Hispanics, and Alaskan Indian and Native American bore during COVID (Bibbins-Domingo, 2020). There appears to be an ever-present connection linking these disparate outcomes with the high rates of underlying conditions and compromised social determinants experienced by these groups. Bibbins-Domingo (2020) explicitly outlined how the social determinants of health intersect with the COVID disparities we witnessed:

> Minority populations are more likely to be exposed to the virus because they are overrepresented in the low-wage, essential workforce at the front lines, including low-wage health care workers who often move between clinics, hospitals, and nursing homes to make a living, thereby magnifying their risk. Poor communities may face challenges implementing social distancing because of housing density and overcrowding, and minority populations are overrepresented in congregate settings, such as homeless shelters and prisons, that increase exposure risk. Minority communities may be more susceptible to severe forms of COVID-19 because of existing disparities in underlying conditions known to be associated with COVID-19 mortality, including hypertension, cardiovascular disease, kidney disease, and diabetes. Although largely preventable or amenable to medical management, these chronic conditions are more common, less likely to be controlled, and more likely to occur at younger ages in these communities. Health care access is also a probable contributor to COVID-19 mortality given the limited availability of both testing and treatments. Much of the testing for severe acute respiratory syndrome coronavirus 2 (SARS-CoV-2) has occurred in the context of a health care evaluation, resulting in barriers for those without insurance. (p. 234)

During COVID, digital inequity was brought into the spotlight when individuals had to rely on technology to make appointments, to access services, to attend school and other health/social service appointments, to seek employment, and to obtain vaccinations. This form of inequity includes lack of access to Internet service or to reliable Internet, interconnectedness to the Internet, lack of high-speed Internet (broadband), and limited digital/technological literacy (Office of Policy Development and Research, 2016a). The plight of digital inequity faced by those who are socioeconomically vulnerable, minoritized populations, and urban/rural communities has been known for its ability to further exacerbate other inequities given the importance of Internet connection as a tool for opportunity and as a resource for information (Office of Policy Development and Research, 2016b).

Life expectancy, which is "the average number of years a newborn can be expected to live based on prevailing age-specific mortality rates (Dubay et al., 2017, p. 4)" is another concerning disparity. Variation in life expectancy across state, regions, and race are correlated by health behaviors, physical and social environment, socioeconomic status, and health system (Dubay et al., 2017). In the United States, there was a decrease in life expectancy from 78.85 years in 2019 to 76.44 years in 2021, equating to a loss of 2.41 years which were "highly racialized" (Masters et al., 2022). Masters et al. (2022) found that "largest losses over the two-year period (2019–2021), occurred in "Non-Hispanic American Indians/Alaskan Natives, Hispanic, and Non-Hispanic Black populations clearly experienced much larger losses in life expectancy than did the non-Hispanic White population. These patterns reflect a long history of systemic racism and its attendant injustices and inadequacies in how the pandemic was managed in the United States (p. 4)."

Pre-pandemic, lower life expectancy was already evident along lines of race which are directly aligned with zip code and along census tract. This divide shows that those who live in certain neighborhoods which are predominantly Black and Brown, poor and environmentally challenged, tend to have lower life expectancy than those who live in more affluent sections of communities. Furthermore, much of this divides parallel lines of segregation, redlining, and urban planning decisions that have impacted placement of highway overpasses, factories, and grocery stores, which also show. The 2019 study series by the Center for Society on Health at Virginia Commonwealth University documented "a 17-year gap in life expectancy across census tracts and identified 15 "islands of disadvantage," neighborhoods where residents face harsh living conditions (p. 3)." Their series exposed 400 years of historical contributors (exclusion from freedom, homeownership, jobs, and civil liberty) to demonstrate that these gaps are not accidental; in fact they are intentional "products of history."

When health disparities are situated in the historical context of exclusion from opportunity, resources, and inequity, this no longer is perplexing. There is an over-accumulation of disparity that is disproportionately carried by the same recurring subset of the population which shows up in their diminished health status. Justice in health exposes the context at the root to illuminate, reconcile, and remediate. A radical and rapid course correction must happen, and it must be ignited to happen. Healthcare providers are obligated to lead this charge because they are in the business of health, they are eyewitnesses to the plight of the most vulnerable, and they are the obvious starting point for change. Justice in health advocates for active reconciliation of the past while moving in a direction that is responsive to the pressing needs and conditions of the present starting with our own profession.

2.3   Reconciling the Past

Several healthcare organizations and professional associations are beginning to attempt to reconcile their troubled racial history with acknowledgments of racism and racist practices which have contributed to health inequity and disparities. These organizations are attempting to move toward more actionable objectives that center racial justice and prioritize health equity. The centering of both health equity and racial justice are necessary pursuits that must happen synergistically given their inextricable interconnectedness. Health equity means "that everyone has a fair and just opportunity to attain their full health potential and that no one is disadvantaged, excluded, or dismissed from achieving this potential. Health equity is the absence of avoidable, unfair, or remediable differences among groups of people, whether those groups are defined by race/ethnicity, culture, class, national origin, or other means of stratification. Many people live at the intersection of identities like race or ethnicity, disability, immigration status, or socioeconomic status. Across these many factors, race and ethnicity often exert the greatest and most consistent measurable impact on the unfair and unjust health outcomes we see" (Aboelata et al., 2020, p. 3).

Although diversity and inclusion terminology and approaches have been used as the "all encapsulating" narrative for equity, traditionally it has rarely built enough momentum to move beyond the aspirational. In spring of 2021, the Centers for Disease Control and Prevention launched a racism and health initiative to demonstrate their commitment "tackling racism as an obstacle to health equity" squarely positioning racism as a public health issue (http://www.cdc.gov/healthequity/racism-disparities/index.htm). The Centers for Disease Control and Prevention views racism as both interpersonal and structural, defined as a "system—consisting of structures, policies, practices, and norms—that assigns value and determines opportunity based on the way people look or the color of their skin. This results in conditions that unfairly advantage some and disadvantage others throughout society ((http://www.cdc.gov/healthequity/racsim-disparities/index.htm)." In response to the national mood demanding accountability and authentic change, several healthcare organizations, institutions, and professional associations have released statements about or calls to action to address racism and health inequity in our society and within the profession.

In the height of the social and moral unrest, the American Academy of Nursing released their report on health equity and racism. The report reflects critical conversion on Health Equity and Racism held in October of 2020 by the American Academy of Nursing Institute for Nursing Leadership intended to stimulate diverse dialogue. Within the report, there are reflections which provide key takeaways, proposed action steps, summaries of panel discussions, and final thoughts. Highlights from the report include its attention to action steps across various nursing setting (clinical, academia, research, policy, and in future conversations). Panelist presented critical touchpoints and calls to action that instill accountability and change leadership which is best culminated by the following quote:

> If you are not in the process of developing action plans for the tables at which you sit as nurses and nurse leaders, then you're not helping the cause (p. 4).

The Future of Nursing 2020–2030: Charting a Path to Achieve Health Equity published by the National Academies of Sciences, Engineering and Medicine (2021) is another profession report that has also been recently released that addressed the nursing response to helping our nation achieve health equity. It identifies a framework that outlines areas for strengthening nursing which impact the social and structural determinants of health that then can lead to improving health equity. The report accentuates the major role that the nursing profession plays in achieving health equity given their positionality across settings where they engage with multiple populations and the holistic approach of their profession. It identifies many aspects of nurses' abilities to work cross-sectorally, engaging with individuals and communities to address root causes of health disparities, and their roles as social innovators, advocates, and system leaders. In light of the current context laden with increasing health disparities, racism, and diminishing health outcomes for the most marginalized and vulnerable, its authors lament that:

> For too long, the United States has overinvested in treating illness and underinvested in promoting health and preventing disease. The nation has spent more on medical care than any other high-income country, yet it has seen consistently worse health outcomes than those of its peer countries, including the lowest life expectancy, more chronic health conditions, and the highest rates of infant mortality. At the same time, the COVID-19 pandemic has starkly revealed Americans' unequal access to opportunities to live a healthy life, often resulting from entrenched structural and systemic barriers that include poverty, racism, and discrimination. These two phenomena—suboptimal health outcomes and inequities in health and health care—are not unrelate. (National Academies of Sciences, Engineering and Medicine, 2021, p. 3).

Given this context and situatedness of the nursing profession as a whole, the academy views nursing as an ideal response to make meaningful strides to advance health equity. The opportunity for the nursing profession to lead in the achievement of health equity is examined critical across areas where nursing can be strengthened (workforce, leadership, education, well-being, and emergency preparedness) to be able to do so.

Other healthcare providers are also responding to the increased urgency of the moment by being explicit in their efforts to acknowledge the interconnectedness of health equity and racial justice with the intention to address both. In the fall of 2021, the American Medical Association (AMA) announced the roll out of their new 3-year organizational strategic plan to embed racial justice and advance health equity 2021–2023 (https://www.ama-assn.org/delivering-care/health-equity/ama-racism-threat-public-health; https://www.ama-assn.org/system/files/2021-05/ama-equity-strategic-plan.pdf). In introducing this strategy, the American Medical Association identified that it "recognizes that racism negatively impacts and exacerbates health inequities among historically marginalized communities. Without systemic and structural-level change, health inequities will continue to exist, and the overall health of the nation will suffer" (https://www.ama-assn.org/delivering-care/health-equity/ama-racism-threat-public-health). This recognition fueled the establishment of an American Medical Association Center of Health Equity (circa 2019) which produced a strategy anchored in critical beliefs about equity-centered solutions. The American Medical Association's Organizational Strategic Plan to Embed Racial Justice and Advance Health Equity, 2021–2023 (https://www.ama-assn.org/system/files/2021-05/ama-equity-strategic-plan.pdf, p. 6) recommends equity-centered solutions include, and are not limited to:

- Ending segregated health care that is reinforced by payer exclusion.
- Establishing national healthcare equity and racial justice standards, benchmarks,incentives, and metrics.
- Ending the use of race-based clinical decision models (including calculators).
- Ensuring that augmented intelligence (AI) is free from harmful, biased algorithms.
- Eliminating all forms of discrimination, exclusion, and oppression in medical and physician education, training, hiring, matriculation, and promotion supported by:

- Mandatory antiracism, structural competency, and equity-explicit training and competencies for all trainees and staff.
- Publicly reported equity assessments for medical schools and hospitals.

- Preventing exclusion of and ensuring just representation of Black, Indigenous, and Latinx people in medical school admissions as well as medical school and hospital leadership ranks.
- Ensuring equity in innovation, including design, development, implementation, and dissemination along with supporting equitable innovation opportunities and entrepreneurship.
- Solidifying connections and coordination between health care and public health.
- Acknowledging and repairing past harms committed by institutions.

Even private citizen and non-healthcare entity stakeholders are also entering the dialogue arena to call for action to advance health equity and truly address health disparities. *The Color of Care* documentary (May 2022), which aired May 1, 2022 (https://www.smithsonianmag.com/videos/category/The_Color_of_Care/), had tones of this same sentiment. This documentary (www.thecolorofcare.org) "traces the origins of racial health disparities to practices that began during slavery in the U.S. and continue today. Using personal testimony, expert interviews, and disturbing data" (p. 4). They provide an important discussion guide to help unpack the film's revelation and provide critical questions and resources as useful education tools for helping to engage around the facts of race and health disparities in the United States (www.thecolorofcare.org). This film provides important evidence-based information that reiterated that racial inequities research and community mobilization efforts can support the reconstruction of knowledge and thought leadership for change. It highlighted what many of us who toil in the sphere of health care that health care is inequitable and unjust. The documentary provided a lens to the pronounced disparities suffered by Black and Brown people in the United States by hearing their stories and lived experiences of blatant racist practices they and their family members endured seeking care. It also contextualized the history of racism in medicine in parallel to the experiences that these communities still suffer today. The documentary exposes and educates providing supplementary resources to further knowledge and facilitate dialogue about this issue.

Table 2.1 highlights these and other recent position documents set forth by healthcare networks, stakeholders, and professional associations. Although not exhaustive, the table offers a snapshot of the budding trajectory of plans to confront racism and advance health equity.

2.4 Strategies for Combating Racism in Health Care

Many of these reports and action papers were created at the height of the disturbing injustices that spurred national reckoning on race and trigger health system actors to reevaluate their own practices and find ways to make change. Each system is at

Table 2.1 Healthcare plans to confront racism and advance health equity

Organization	Document	Document link
Future of Nursing	The future of nursing 2020–2030: Charting a path to achieve health equity[13]	https://www.nationalacademies.org/event/05-11-2021/the-future-of-nursing-2020-2030-charting-a-path-to-achieve-health-equity-report-release-webinar Summary: Addresses the nursing response to helping our nation achieve health equity. It identifies a framework that outlines areas for strengthening nursing which impact the social and structural determinants of health that then can lead to improving health equity. Areas that are discussed where nursing can be strengthened include workforce, leadership, education, Well-being, and emergency preparedness
Prevention Institute	Building bridges: The strategic imperative for advancing health equity and racial justice[14]	https://www.preventioninstitute.org/publications/building-bridges-strategic-imperative-advancing-health-equity-and-racial-justice Summary: This paper illuminates the interrelatedness of health equity and racial justice. It provides principle and parameters for understanding the intersection of health equity and racial justice and raises insights on the tensions within this understanding. Two equity frameworks are offered to help understand equity as a process from various dimensions and strategic opportunities to advance this work are laid out
American Academy of Nursing Institute for Nursing Leadership	A critical conversation on health equity and racism[15]	https://www.aannet.org/initiatives/institute-for-nursing-leadership/2020report Summary: This report offers reflections, key takeaways, proposed action steps, summaries of panel discussions, and final thoughts. Highlights from the report include its attention to action steps across various nursing setting (clinical, academia, research, policy, and in future conversations). Panelist presented critical touchpoints and calls to action that instill accountability and change leadership

(continued)

Table 2.1 (continued)

Organization	Document	Document link
American Medical Association	Organizational strategic plan to embed racial justice and advance health equity 2021–2023[12]	https://www.ama-assn.org/system/files/2021-05/ama-equity-strategic-plan.pdf Summary: This plan is a 3-year roadmap that serves to provide strategic direction to the associations' achievement of health equity and justice through action and accountability. It entails five key strategic approaches to (1) embed racial and social justice throughout the AMA enterprise culture, systems, policies, and practices; (2) build alliances and share power with historically marginalized and minority physicians and other stakeholders; (3) push upstream to address all determinants of health and the root causes of inequities; (4) ensure equitable structures sand opportunities in innovation; and (5) foster pathways for truth, racial healing, reconciliation, and transformation for AMA's past (p. 8–9). The report provides robust definitions, discusses facilitators of organizational change, actions and accountability, and 12 appendices
World Innovation Summit for Health	Nurses for health equity guidelines for tackling the social determinants of health[16]	Nurses for Health Equity: Guidelines for Tackling the Social Determinants of Health (PDF) Summary: This technical report (2021) outlines the need for expedited investment in nursing as the approach to address health equity and the social determinants of health. In the report there are six key domains of focus that include education and training; research and evaluation; clinical practice and community impact; health system and organizations; partnership; and advocacy
The Smithsonian Channel and Harpo Productions	The color of care	www.thecolorofcare.org Summary: It is a documentary chronologically tracing racial inequity in health care that includes personal accounts and the lived experiences of community members and healthcare providers. The site also provides discussion and educational material to accompany the film for use with students, community members, and organizations

various stages and phases of this work which has become accelerated and trigger many to seek concrete solutions that can respond now with the appropriate amounts of rigor and expediency. The Prevention Institute's 2020 paper illuminating the interrelatedness of health equity and racial justice provides principles and parameters for understanding this intersection and offers a strategic imperative for advancing both (Aboelata et al., 2020). Within this strategic imperative are five recommended actions to advance health equity and racial justice. The first identifies the need to align our data and data analysis within a blended framework of racial justice and health equity. This approach brings historical and present-day drivers of each into the forefront, allowing a clearer picture to identify most impactful measures which enhances strategies and outcomes for all. Second, they raise the importance of naming racially patterned inequities in our communications about health equities by framing the convergence of the issues of racial justice and health equity. A third recommendation is cross-sector collaboration which will increase impact, resources, and capacities to deal with health equity and racial justice, while helping each organization benefit from new knowledge that can enhance their own culture. Fourth, system and structural change in addition to critical community organizing to transform power are key strategies for achieving health equity and racial justice. And finally, the recommendation for transformative resource allocation and investments to catalyze infrastructure and opportunity investment in the most marginalized communities.

Of equal importance in attaining a convergent approach to health equity and health justice is to attend to confront racism in health care. Hostetter and Klein (2021) have proposed various approaches to help overcome the ongoing issues of racism in health care. Proposed are exemplars of university medical centers who have found unique and interesting ways to start addressing this issue. The authors consolidated approaches used by some institutions into the following list of strategies:

– Examining institutional policies with an equity lens.
– Establishing accountability frameworks such as equity score cards.
– Auditing medical school curricula for erroneous references to race.
– Reviewing clinical algorithms that erroneously rely on race.
– Investing in scholarships for students of color interest in health professions.
– Training leadership and staff in diversity, equity, inclusion, and antiracism principles.
– Creating real-time reporting initiatives to track and respond to racist or other discriminatory behavior.
– Reviewing vendor relationships to support Black and other minority-owned businesses.
– Creating more equitable workplaces, including efforts to build wealth and opportunities for advancement.
– Listening to and learning form patients and healthcare professionals of color.

(Hostetter & Klein, 2021, p. 3)

2.5   Conclusion

A health apartheid exists in America where there are clear chasms of inequity that are predicated on racial lines. Health is the one of the most egregious areas of them all, because it is the center of the human experience, the right to which has been endowed to us all. It is a professional, moral, and ethical affront to the very ideal of health and the practice of health care.

"We can't achieve health equity without racial justice, and we can't achieve racial justice without health equity" (Aboelata et al., 2020, p. 14). These equity issues are intersecting and require a justice in health approach which overcomes the inclination to separate and silo. Instead, justice in health moves toward redressing inequity by integrating this interconnected web of issues into all education and training of healthcare providers, into all structures (policies, procedures, and practices) and into all research. Health justice acts with the acknowledgment of the deeply rooted historical context that still shapes inequities and determines health.

2.6   Reflective Questions and Considerations

1. What information about the history of health was new information and how do you think that it has impacted the health of communities?
2. How do we start to overcome the history of health today? What steps can you and your institution take to help make this happen? What are the barriers to making it happen?
3. What structural changes need to happen to make meaningful changes in closing the gaps in health disparities?

References

Aboelata, M., Rivas, R., Williams, L., & Yañezin, E. (2020). *Building bridges: The strategic imperative for advancing health equity and racial justice a concept paper prepared by prevention institute*. Retrieved from: https://www.preventioninstitute.org/publications/building-bridges-strategic-imperative-advancing-health-equity-and-racial-justice

American Association of Colleges of Nursing. (2021). *AACN fact sheet: Enhancing diversity in the nursing workforce*. Retrieved August 31, 2021, from https://www.aacnnursing.org/News-Information/Fact-Sheets/Enhancing-Diversity

American Medical Association. (2021). *Organizational strategic plan to embed racial justice and advance equity 2021–2023*. Retrieved from: https://www.ama-assn.org/system/files/2021-05/ama-equity-strategic-plan.pdf

Anachebe (2021) from Article: Now is the time to diversity the nation's medical workforce. April 12, 2021 (Brookings). https://www.brookings.edu/blog/how-we-rise/2021/04/12/now-is-the-time-to-diversify-the-nations-medical-workforce-heres-how

Arnett, M. J., Thorpe, R. J., Gaskin, D. J., Bowie, J. V., & LaVeist, T. A. (2016). Race, medical mistrust, and segregation in primary care as usual source of care: Findings from the exploring health disparities in integrated communities study. *Journal of Urban Health, 93*(3), 456–467.

Association of American Medical Colleges. (2018). *Figure 18. Percentage of all active physicians by race/ethnicity, 2018*. Retrieved August 31, 2022, from https://www.aamc.org/data-reports/workforce/interactive-data/figure-18-percentage-all-active-physicians-race/ethnicity-2018

Bibbins-Domingo, K. (2020). This time must be different: disparities during the COVID-19 pandemic. *Annals of Internal Medicine, 173*(3), 233–234.

Blanchard, S. A., Rivers, R., Martinez, W., & Agodoa, L. (2021). Building the network of minority health research investigators: A novel program to enhance leadership and success of underrepresented minorities in biomedical research. *Ethnicity & Disease, 29*(Suppl 1), 119–122. https://doi.org/10.18865/ed.29.S1.119

Borrero, S., Zite, N., & Creinin, M. D. (2012). Federally funded sterilization: Time to rethink policy? *American Journal of Public Health, 102*(10), 1822–1825.

Byrd, W. M., & Clayton, L. A. (2001). Race, medicine, and health care in the United States: A historical survey. *Journal of the National Medical Association, 93*(3 Suppl), 11S.

Castillo, R. J., & Guo, K. L. (2011). A framework for cultural competence in health care organizations. *Health Care Management, 30*(3), 205–214. https://doi.org/10.1097/HCM.0b013e318225dfe6

Center for Society and Health. (2019). *Health equity in Northern Virginia*. Retrieved July 2, 2022, from https://societyhealth.vcu.edu/work/the-projects/health-equity-in-northern-virginia.html

Clayborne, E. P., Martin, D. R., Goett, R. R., Chandrasekaran, E. B., & McGreevy, J. (2021, January 2). Diversity pipelines: The rationale to recruit and support minority physicians. *Journal of American Collage Emergency Physicians Open, 2*(1), e12343. https://doi.org/10.1002/emp2.12343. PMCID: PMC7823093.

Cornely, P. B. (1956). Segregation and discrimination in medical care in the United States. *American Journal of Public Health and the Nation's Health, 46*(9), 1074–1081.

Dula, A. (1994). African American suspicion of the healthcare system is justified: What do we do about it? *Cambridge Quarterly of Healthcare Ethics, 3*(3), 347–357.

Goode, C. A., & Landefeld, T. (2018). The lack of diversity in healthcare. *Journal of Best Practices in Health Professions Diversity, 11*(2), 73–95.

Highet, M. J. (2005). Body snatching & grave robbing: Bodies for science. *History and Anthropology, 16*(4), 415–440.

Hostetter, M. & Klein, S. (2021, October 18). *Confronting racism in health Care: Moving from proclamations to new practices*. Commonwealth Fund. Retrieved May 3, 2022, from www.commonwealthfund.org/publications/2021/oct/confrontin-racism-health-care

Howard Hughes Medical Center. (2022). *HHMI Program*. Retrieved June 28, 2022, from https://www.hhmi.org/news/new-hhmi-program-pledges-1-5-billion-early-career-faculty-committed-diversity-equity-inclusion

Jones, M., & Saines, M. (2019). The eighteen of 1918-1919: Black nursed and the great flu pandemic in the United States. *American Journal of Public Health, 109*(6), 877–882.

Kendrick, K., Withey, S., Batson, A., Wright, S. M., & O'Rourke, P. (2020). Predictors of satisfying and impactful clinical shadowing experiences for underrepresented minority high school students interested in healthcare careers. *Journal of the National Medical Association, 112*(4), 381–386.

Kennedy, B. R., Mathis, C. C., & Woods, A. K. (2007). African Americans and their distrust of the health care system: Healthcare for diverse populations. *Journal of Cultural Diversity, 14*(2), 56–60.

Largent, E. A. (2018). Public health, racism, and the lasting impact of hospital segregation. *Public Health Reports, 133*(6), 715–720.

Masters, K., Aron, L., & Woolf, S. (2022). *Changes in life expectancy between 2019 and 2021 in The United States and 21 peer countries Rxiv*. 2022.04.05.22273393. https://doi.org/10.1101/2022.04.05.22273393.

National Academies of Sciences, Engineering, and Medicine. (2021). *The future of nursing 2020–2030: Charting a path to achieve health equity*. The National Academies Press. https://doi.org/10.17226/25982

Ndugga and Atria (2021). Retrieved from: Disparities in Health and Health Care: 5 Key Questions and Answers – Issue Brief – 8396-05 | KFF (https://www.kff.org/report-section/disparities-in-health-and-health-care-5-keyquestions-and-answers-issue-brief/) .

Nieblas-Bedolla, E. M. P. H., Christophers, B., Nkinsi, N. T., Schumann, P. D., & Stein, E. (2020, December). Changing how race is portrayed in medical education: Recommendations from medical students. *Academic Medicine, 95*(12), 1802–1806. https://doi.org/10.1097/ACM.0000000000003496

Owens, D. C., & Fett, S. M. (2019). Black maternal and infant health: Historical legacies of slavery. *American Journal of Public Health, 109*(10), 1342–1345.

Reilly, P. R. (1987). Involuntary sterilization in the United States: A surgical solution. *The Quarterly Review of Biology, 62*(2), 153–170.

Reilly, P. R. (2015). Eugenics and involuntary sterilization: 1907–2015. *Annual Review of Genomics and Human Genetics, 16*, 351–368.

Rivera-Nieves, J., & Abreu, M. T. (2013). A call for investment in education of US minorities in the 21st century. *Gastroenterology, 144*(5), 863–867. https://doi.org/10.1053/j.gastro.2013.03.020

Rosa, W. E., Hannaway, C. J., McArdle, C., McManus, M. F., Alharahsheh, S. T., & Marmot, M. (2021). *Nurses for health equity: Guidelines for tackling the social determinants of health.* World Health Innovation Summit for Health (WISH). Retrieved from: https://www.wish.org. qa/reports/nurses-for-health-equity-guidelines-for-tackling-the-social-determinants-of-health/

Saizan, A. L., Douglas, A., Elbuluk, N., & Taylor, S. (2021). A diverse nation calls for a diverse healthcare force. *EClinical Medicine, 34*. https://doi.org/10.1016/j.eclinm.2021.100846

Savitt, T. L. (1982). The use of blacks for medical experimentation and demonstration in the old south. *The Journal of Southern History, 48*(3), 331–348.

The Smithsonian Channel and Harpo Productions. (2022). *The color of care.* Retrieved from: www.thecolorofcare.org

The United States Government. Office of Policy Development and Research. (2016a). Community Development and the Digital Divide. *Evidence Matters.* Retrieved July 11, 2022, from https:// www.huduser.gov/portal/periodicals/em/fall16/highlight1.html

The United States Government. Office of Policy Development and Research. (2016b). Digital inequality and low-income households. *Evidence matters.* Retrieved July 11, 2022, from https://www.huduser.gov/portal/periodicals/em/fall16/highlight2.html

Thomas, S. B., & Quinn, S. C. (1991). The Tuskegee Syphilis Study, 1932 to 1972: Implications for HIV education and AIDS risk education programs in the black community. *American Journal of Public Health, 81*(11), 1498–1505.

Tobbell, D., & D'Antonio, P. (2022). *National Commission to address racism in nursing: The history of racism in nursing: A review of existing scholarship.* Retrieved from: https://www. nursingworld.org/~49b97e/globalassets/practiceandpolicy/workforce/commission-to-address-racism/racism-in-nursing-report-series.pdf

Varma, R. (2018). U.S. Science and engineering workforce: Underrepresentation of women and minorities. *American Behavioral Scientist, 00*(0), 1–6. https://doi.org/10.1177/ 000276421876884

Whitla, D. K., Orfield, G., Silen, W., Teperow, C., Howard, C., & Reede, J. (2003, May). Educational benefits of diversity in medical school. *Academic Medicine, 78*(5), 460–466.

Witzig, R. (1996). The medicalization of race: Scientific legitimization of a flawed social construct. *Annals of Internal Medicine, 125*(8), 675–679.

Wolf, S. T., Jablonski, N. G., & Kenney, W. L. (2020). Examining "race" in physiology. *American Journal of Physiology-Heart and Circulatory Physiology, 319*(6), H1409–H1413.

Woolf, S. H., Aron, L., Chapman, D. A., Dubay, L., Zimmerman, E., Snellings, L. C., Hall, L., Haley, A. D., Holla, N., Ayers, K., Lowenstein, C., & Waidmann, T. A. (2017). *Center on Society and Health, Virginia Commonwealth University, and Urban Institute. The health of the states report. Spotlight on life expectancy and mortality.* Retrieved July 2, 2022, from https:// societyhealth.vcu.edu/media/society-health/pdf/HOTS_Supplement2_FINAL.pdf

Chapter 3
Frameworks for Framing Justice in Health

This chapter is deeply philosophical and driven by the introduction and exploration of key theories most critical to meet the health and well-being challenges we face as a nation. Highlighted are discussions of critical theories and perspectives that include but are not limited to postcolonial and emancipatory inquiry, social justice in nursing practice, structural violence, and structural justice. Discussion about the social determinants of health are at the forefront to help introduce the reader to contextual causes that determine health guided by these various theoretical perspectives. This chapter serves to synthesize structural and root causes through exposing the hidden realities of power, privilege, and social identity.

3.1 Introduction

There is a place for history, theory, and evidence to guide exploration and understanding of our experiences. The coupling of experiences (past and present) with the translation of knowledge (evidence and theory) provides information to influence and inform action. Applying theoretical and historical perspectives have traditionally been an indelible part of the academic process of empirical inquiry. In the healthcare profession, theory is fundamental and foundational to grounding our practice and underutilized in seeking solutions.

Theory accentuates a unique lens that sheds light on a particular phenomenon by sharing perspectives from past and present insights to explain conditions and circumstances. Many healthcare theorists engage in narratives highlighting the provision of care and what is perceived by the profession to be important practices, skills, and values to be upheld by their particular specialty. As the conditions determining health became more pronounced, theories from various disciplines were integrated to shed light on the human condition and its circumstances.

Critical frameworks have continued to emerge as instrumental in examining the current health context and illuminating the complex health conditions that negatively affect health outcomes among disparate populations. Determining which orientation and paradigms are best suited for this task should ensure that at a minimum they embody two important components. The first being that it is action-oriented and action driven and second that it embraces ecological thinking with an astuteness for structural drivers and redressing root causes.

Examination of solutions to rectify these real and present threats to well-being requires immediate action and structural reconciliation to ameliorate them. Critical perspectives and orientations are astutely attuned to the visible and hidden realities of the human condition and sit in solidarity with doing the hard work of making change often in unpopular and difficult spaces.

3.2 Critical Theory

Critical theory has a long-standing tradition as a responsive voice of the oppressed and abject register of dominant systems of power, oppression, injustice, and inequity. It has been defined as "adequate only if it meets three criteria: it must be explanatory, practical, and normative, all at the same time. That is, it must explain what is wrong with current social reality, identify the actors to change it, and provide both clear norms for criticism and achievable practical goals for social transformation" (Bohman, 2005, p. 1). To be critical is to be cognizant of our taken for granted assumptions of the larger world context and speaking truth to power about its dysfunctional functions. Criticalness confronts, disrupts, and unpacks by bringing to the forefront that which has typically been in the background. It refocuses with a transparency and truth that centers the reality of historically excluded and marginalized populations (such as marginalized, racialized, LGBTQIA+, the disabled, etc.) as intersecting and one which matters.

The critical paradigm elucidates history to expose the often-hidden realities of disparate populations to provide evidence of truth and validation of their experiences and shed light on the root causes of those experiences. Shedding light is fundamental to liberation of the human condition which is what critical theory seeks to achieve and democracy is seen as the seat of freedom and justice where transformation can happen. Critical examination acknowledges upfront that inequity exists due to the inequitable distribution of power, privilege, race, bias, and structured oppression of the powerless. Through approaches grounded in critical consciousness of these realities, critical examination asks the unasked questions and disrupts dominant discourses to illuminate the root. Critical inquiry is not what we want to see but what truly lies beneath many of the issues we identify as inequitable and unjust.

Social inquiry is at the root of critical theory, a tradition that grew out of German philosophers from the Frankfurt School from Horkheimer and Adorno, Marcuse, to Habermas (Corradetti, 2012; McLaughlin, 1999). Critical theorists then and now seek to expose the human condition in an effort to emancipate it. Critical theory is derived from a core focus on the dialectic between the human being in relation to the society (social reality), deemed as exploitive and inhumane. Critical traditions evolved from being a theory of society to one that encapsulates a multiplicity of traditions such as humanism, colonialism, intersectionality, feminism, structuralism, and emancipatory inquiry. Its lens is skewed toward matters of justice and power and their interaction with class, gender, race, religion, and institutions (Patton, 2002). The tendency of critical paradigm is to illuminate and denounce to instigate action that leads to human emancipation. Central to understanding the ideals of human emancipation were the theories, interrogation of democracy, ideology, and communicative action.

Within the critical tradition democracy is a space that makes human liberation and emancipation attainable. Ideology is a constraint of this possibility because it stifles the pursuit of the normative of truth and justice by distorting communication which undermines how democracy occurs and its processes (Bohman, 2005). It "masks consciousness" (Lutz et al., 1997) and is used to serve at the will of transient purposes and intentions. Communicative action attends to the use of knowledge and language as mechanisms where power is reproduced through rules and order of communication to reify and institutionalize norms. Understanding the present contextualized reality full of tradition, ideology, and orders of political and social life to enact change is of great concern to critical theorists. Critical theory has been the foundation to understanding and interpreting society and its situated knowledge which is viewed as political and interdiscursive. In doing so, critical theory analyzes society and its knowledge interdependently, and theory is a part of the knowingness; hence critical theory becomes reflective of itself in the process. Devetak (2005) reminds us that "the purpose underlying critical, as opposed to traditional, conceptions of theory is to improve human existence by abolishing injustice" (Horkheimer, 1972). As articulated by Horkheimer (1972, p. 215), this conception of theory does not simply present an expression of the "concrete historical situation"; it also acts as "a force within [that situation] to stimulate change (p. 165)." This theory moves away from an objective reality that separates the individual from its context, values from facts, and subject from object to examine unexamined assumptions necessary to achieve social and political transformation.

3.3   Critical Perspectives

Aligned with this critical theoretical orientation are perspectives which have been influenced and/or shaped by critical theoretical underpinnings. Emancipatory inquiry is the intersection (praxis) of theory and action where harmful practices and ideology are illuminated to actuate human freedom. Praxis, according to Hoggan et al. (2017), entails "a specific type of epistemic break: a rupture which involves a double movement of critical negation and creative exploration". This critical distance allows individual and collective subjects to deepen their rational understanding of the structural forces which give rise to the order of things. Through this activity, we can then begin to identify possibilities for action that increase human well-being. This often—but not always—necessitates an explicit rejection and critique of dominant ideologies and social relations which unnecessarily harm or hinder human development (p. 57). While the goal of critical orientation is that of emancipation, there are distinct ways to achieve this based on the perspective. Critical social traditionalists view praxis as the point of reflective action obtained when movement from false to critical consciousness is enabled. On the other hand, hermeneutic philosophers within the critical tradition embrace praxis as the "understanding of shared meanings, not critique of power and oppression, that one gains a more sensitized understanding of another's life world" (Lutz et al., 1997, p. 25). Both understand that emancipation is required to counteract structures of oppression and exploitation, and therefore the moral obligation of the philosopher is to think and to act (Lutz et al., 1997). Any movement into such realms of emancipatory understanding will cause important and necessary discomfort. To pursue "an inquiry of discomfort" is to "identify and promote a beneficial shift from dualistic, categorical, and entrenched subjective positionality to a more ambiguous engagement with social reality" that is transformative (Wolgemuth & Donohue, 2006, p. 1024).

3.3.1   Critical Race Theory

With critical awareness and deep understanding comes transformation of individuals and societies that spur intellectual, social, and political movements. We see this unfolding in real time with the surge of wokeness into new dimensions of knowledge and consciousness generated through critical race theory. The issues of structural racism, discrimination, and oppression that are illuminated by critical race theory are not new. There are literally centuries of historical evidential shoulders that this theory stands upon. Critical race theory exposes the myth of neutrality and exposes institutions, systems, and its policies as inherently embedding and reifying societal biases, power imbalances, discrimination, and the reproduction of racial hierarchy. One of the most interesting and cogent articulation of this founding premise of critical race theory is explained as follows:

> …Indeed the appearance of neutrality primarily operated to obscure the fact that the perspective of the white majority is embedded within this view. In addition, the concept of discrimination is so limited that the remedies for it cannot adequately recognize all forms of discrimination nor overcome the continuing effect that it has had on our society. In a 1978 article, which legal scholars of color found to be one of the best written critical legal studies pieces, Alan Freeman pointed out that the view of racism and racial oppression embedded in traditional legal thinking is that of the perpetrators of racial oppression as opposed to its victims. In a 1978 article, Charles Lawrence noted that the Supreme Court's decision of race discrimination as the product of consciously racially motivated decision making is inadequate because it overlooks the impact if unconscious forms of racism. Derrick Bell's interest in convergence principle and racial realism went a step beyond Lawrence. In his interest convergence principle, Bell asserted that blacks only make substantial progress against racial oppression when their interests align with those of white elites. From this interest convergence principle comes Bell's racial realism—that racism is an integral, permanent, and indestructible part of American society (Brown & Jackson, 2013, p. 14)

These origins that challenge inherent neutrality of all system, structures, and policies made way for the social discourse of race as part of and not separate from structures. Crenshaw (2010), one of its early and widely respected leading scholars, identifies critical race theory not as a definition but as a "socio-cultural narrative." Crenshaw posits that CRT "is not so much an intellectual unit filled with natural stuff-theories, themes, practices, and the like-but one that is dynamically constituted by a series of contestations and convergences pertaining to the ways that racial power is understood and articulated in the post-civil rights era" (Crenshaw, 2010, p. 1261) and "that it provides a particularly robust prism for engaging today's "post-racialism" (Crenshaw, 2010, p. 1261). Crenshaw (1991) has also illuminated the theory of intersectionality that points to the role multiple identities (woman, Black, poor) play in creating intersectional subordination, the layer of vulnerabilities that further compromise well-being and impact outcomes.

Although critical race theory has been generative in its ability to engage a socio-cultural narrative and dynamic dialogue about race, it has been politically polarizing and weaponized as divisive. What it, as other modes of critical inquiry do, is question assumptions, norms, and values about what is and offers perspective that may feel contrary to the constructed reality.

3.3.2   Postcolonial Theory

Postcolonial theory is a critical perception that seeks to unpack historical and culture practices of exploitation, imposed domination, and economic objectification that shape and influence current inequitable conditions. Global colonial expansion of imperialist colonies fueled greed and extraction of resources to obtain and increase wealth. The cost of this was paid for by First Nations populations, Indigenous communities, and slave labor. Many nations around the world are settler colonial societies: "settler colonialism is the process by which a nation "strives for the dissolution of native societies" and "erects a new colonial society on the expropriated land base" (Tobell & D'Antonio, 2022, p. 17). As such, systems of oppression and domination were established within the acts of colonization that are evident and persist today. The aftermath of this structured socio, political, and economic violence is the emergence of an altered consciousness reflected in postcolonial theory. This emergence that is pointedly described by Rukundwa and Van Aarde (2007):

> …In a dislocated culture, postcolonial theory does not declare war on the past, but challenges the consequences of the past that are exploitative. In so doing, postcolonial theory engages the psychology of both the colonised and the coloniser in the process of decolonisation. Those engaged in and those affected by colonisation and imperialism are consciously brought to a level of responsibility, because the cultural revolution refuses to endure a state of subjugation. Postcolonial theory raises self-consciousness which revolutionizes the minds of the colonised and the coloniser to build a new society where liberty and equity prevail (pp. 1189–1190).

The theory reflects on the past to enact justice through acknowledgment and rectification of those subjugated by colonizing forces. This rectification holds to the task of restoration of what was lost (cultural practices, traditions, languages, and customs), while challenging assumed superiority of Western domination and empowering the disempowered (Parsons & Harding, 2011). Postcolonial theory informs our thoughts and actions of health equity by exposing a social justice agenda situated within a global and historical context and narratives.

3.4   Social Justice

Social justice is associated with the critical tradition in its pursuit of a justice and equitable society. Aspirations for a just and equitable society is one where access to privilege, power, and opportunity are universally held by all irrespective of ethnicity, social, or geographical location. It is the pursuit of fairness for those who have been treated unfairly and the realization that there must be actions toward ensuring its achievement. Social justice assumes a basic social order that imposes inequity on the most vulnerable to the benefit of the privileged (Peter, 2018). Therefore, social justice must be enacted to overcome this inequity and equality and… for all.

In health, social justice is upheld as a human right and an ethical imperative of practice. The American Medical Association remarks that "…in the context of health and health care, a commitment to social justice means believing that everyone ought to be able to avoid preventable disease and escape premature death (Patel, 2015, p. 894)." Yet Donohoe and Schiff (2014) identify that:

> …Despite the obvious relevance of social issues to patient health, physicians as a group are not particularly engaged in civic redress of injustice and oppression: more than half of physician organizations are doing little to ameliorate racial and ethnic health disparities (Peek et al., 2012), physicians tend to vote less than members of other social groups (Grande et al., 2007), and, when physicians lobby Congress, their efforts tend to focus on issues that affect them professionally and financially (Gruen et al., 2006), rather than those that affect their patients' health (Donohoe & Schiff, 2014, p. 703).

There are pedagogical ways to train and educate providers in a social justice orientation. This training opportunity has been fueled by the urgent need to address ongoing health disparities and have been echoed in the recent increase of action statements that were illuminated in Chap. 2. A justice in health approach encourages the training of all providers in the system with a social justice orientation throughout all of their curriculum touchpoints and not exclusively within specific course options which usually are community, public, and population health curricula. Every subject that a healthcare student is offered must include both social justice and health equity, even in the biological sciences offerings of pathophysiology, microbiology, etc.

While health professionals have instilled practice competencies and ethical mandates of social justice as part of their practice and aspects of education, others such as nursing originated from social justice beginning as the very foundation and root of practice.

3.4.1 Social Justice and Nursing

Social justice comfortably sits in the critical paradigm and traditions—for some disciplines such as nursing, it has historically been used as the discipline's approach to health practice and act of critical caring. Falk-Rafael (2005) contends that nurses have a moral imperative to re-engage themselves in the roots of their nursing practice which is social justice because they bear witness to individuals and their contextualized conditions. Connecting nurses with the root of their practice helps us to better understand why nurses practice extends beyond one specific type of setting. Nurses practice in schools, in public health departments, in universities, as nurse scientists, as researchers, as policy-makers, and in the community. They are health innovators whose care encompasses the whole person, their families, and the community which come from their historical social justice foundations.

Florence Nightingale is frequently heralded as the mother of nursing—and is often pictured in the corridors of many nursing schools. She is ceremoniously acknowledged in many nursing events from graduation ceremony to professional conferences, always showcased in an early century picture where she is cloaked in iconic nursing regalia of the past. To say Florence is revered in nursing would be an understatement. A lesser celebrated nurse, but equitably formidable nurse leader is Mary Seacole, a British-Jamaican nurse who practiced during the same era—when nursing was being formalized into official practice status during the Crimean War (Baptiste et al., 2021; Staring-Derks et al., 2015).

Both Florence and Mary were nurse leaders with significant practice roles inspired by injustices that they witnessed in the lives of the most vulnerable. These nurses passionately worked to overcome conditions that impacted the health of their patients. Florence's observations let her examine more closely the causes of the sicknesses that affected wounded soldiers. Using information that we now call "data" and approaches that are akin to epidemiological surveillance, she quickly connected the dots that improper sanitation practices were an environmental justice issue because it caused infection and disease (https://en.wikipedia.org/wiki/Florence_Nightingale). She advocated for change of those conditions for her patients knowing that to treat disease without the conditions that create them is futile.

Mary Seacole was an assertive entrepreneurial spirited nurse who used her cultural Jamaican healing practices to serve the British military during the war (Staring-Derks et al., 2015). Although her request to help provide nursing support was initially denied, she was determined to assist and set up her own hotel to provide care (https://www.nationalgeographic.org/article/mary-seacole/; https://en.wikipedia.org/wiki/Mary_Seacole). She attended to the physical and emotional health of the soldiers by taking care of their wounds, feeding them, and providing support at her own expense (https://en.wikipedia.org/wiki/Mary_Seacole). She is a compassionate care worker whose practice was an act of caring and healing. While both Florence and Mary delivered care, beneath the treatment was the attention to the patient, the entirety of their needs, and their determination to act on meeting those needs.

Other notable nurses include abolitionists such as Harriet Tubman (Crewe, 2007) and Sojourner Truth (Patten, 1986) who are more known for their acts of bravery to tackle sobering issues of social justice and humanity (the abolishment of slavery and women rights and suffrage) and less as nurse activists and practitioner (Baptiste et al., 2021). Lillian Wald and Mary Brewster were inner city nurses who established the Henry Street settlement in New York in 1893: a community health program that provided holistic accessible care to the working class and the poor using public health measures (Philips, 1999; Buhler-Wilkerson, 1993). Lillian Wald would be recognized as the founder of public health nursing and establishing its national identity. Nancy Milio formed the Mom and Tots community clinic in Detroit during the 1950s–1970s offering needed services to break down access to healthcare barriers faced by the local under-resourced community (https://news.virginia.edu/content/nursing-forum-explores-what-nancy-milio-s-detroit-mom-and-tots-clinic-did-so-well). These nurses are not anomalies. They are exemplars of the legacy of nursing practice with what Falk-Rafael (2005) calls critical caring.

> Speaking truth to power, that is, influencing public policies that impact health, advocating for those whose voices have been silenced, and challenging ideologies that contribute to the exclusion of some groups for the benefit of others, is to practice empowered caring (Falk-Rafael, 2005, p. 222)

Critical caring is the natural expression that emerges from an ecological understanding of the totality of the human experience and the expectation of healthful conditions that will manifest human flourishing. Human flourishing is a legitimate healthcare goal, and while there will be clients who are able to flourish despite the risks and harms, there are mitigable challenges and structural constraints creating barriers for vulnerable populations and communities. When decisions for care or treatment are being made, it is essential that our determination includes a critical examination of the root issues and causes essential to achieving health for the individuals in the context of their communities (Sellman, 2005). The individual and their context are inseparable which has been repeatedly evidenced by the hemorrhaging of health disparities seen in racialized and minoritized.

When health practice and context intersect, both client and provider come into the knowing of the wholeness of each person. Health decisions and opportunities move in relation to the ecological wellness of the human being at its center. The need for continuity of care is prioritized to start before illness occurs and transcends the clients' own home, throughout hospitalization or clinic visit, to discharge back into their community, similar to a feedback loop. It is the formation of a community of care with shared health equity and health justice values, beliefs, and practices lived and demonstrated. This care structure may require policy and practice changes in the organization of health services, the administration of services, and the education of both clients and their healthcare providers.

> An analogy that I often use to understand the praxis of communal inquiry is playing chess. One can never predict the moves of a chess game in advance of the playing. But to play one must know the rules. It would be pedagogically advantageous to ask ourselves, how do we learn these rules? How do we learn what to do, when, in what context? How do we learn what not to do? How do we learn to regulate our emotions while playing? What roles do the

following play in the acquisition of the capacity to play well: lecturing, modelling, attentive observation, actual playing, and reflection on the playing? It is important to remember that once the first move is made in chess, there is a ritual that is followed in one way or another. Although one can never predict the moves in advance of the playing, one can detect almost somatically when someone has not followed the rules or has made an indiscriminate move. So much more is required than merely knowing the rules. To play chess well one must immerse oneself in the playing of chess and slowly build up an understanding of what moves are advantageous and what moves are foolhardy in a certain context. And the context is never, or very rarely the same. (*Critical and Creative Thinking*, Volume 15, No. 1 2007, p. 7.)

Mary and Florence nursing practice was shaped and refined by the context of the war which spurred a focus on public health well into the twenty-first century. COVID-19, racial injustice, and political unrest too are sharpening our practice and refining our practice context. First, the pandemic has taught us many lessons—perhaps the most paramount being the fractured state and focus of our nation's health and healthcare system. When the pandemic hit, it came as no surprise that the healthcare levees broke. COVID-19 hit communities with the worst health disparities, and highest rates of underlying conditions were the hardest because our system lacked a structured focus on prevention and addressing the root causes that contribute to common underlying conditions.

We can improve our system and health inequities by implementing a coordinated system of care that is both equitable and just—from the community to the hospital—that addresses people's health beyond the absence of disease. Much of this work starts with healthcare reform. The Biden-Harris 1.9 trillion-dollar American Rescue Plan (https://www.whitehouse.gov/american-rescue-plan/) is just the first step on the pathway to desperately needed national health reform. It will fund critical public health investments ranging from health service provision to community health center expansion and beyond—yet really it is just a sobering reminder that both the system and the people need to be rescued. We need a nursing informed rescue plan.

By default, nurses are already positioned in workspaces that can implement change. Nurses work in schools, in public health and social service agencies, in government, in homes, in communities, in research-led science, and community-engaged research. The core of nursing practice has always been in holistic health matters and in particular those crises of basic morality and human dignity such as poverty, racism, and inequity. Historically nurses, who in the face of the most adverse of circumstances such as slavery to wars and infectious diseases, have stood up to oppression, injustice, and inequity. The legacy of nursing includes those prominent figures mentioned earlier: Harriet Tubman (abolitionist/community health), Mary Seacole (public/community health), Sojourner Truth (abolitionist), and Florence Nightingale (environmental justice advocate). They were all instrumental change makers in our nation's health systems, practices, and policies.

Nurses today are still social justice practitioners who are set to lead and affect change on multiple fronts from the environment to infectious disease to social justice. Yet, while nurses make up the largest segment of our nation's healthcare system, their expertise and input continue to be underutilized and overlooked. Like the

American Rescue Plan (https://www.whitehouse.gov/american-rescue-plan/), we need rescue conversations about the reimagining and reevaluation of all of our systems, assumptions, practices, and priorities. Nurses need to be at the table informing and helping to lead these changes that include their thought leadership.

Justice in health comes from the heart of a nurse who believes that nurses have moved too far away from the roots of nursing practice—social justice and that society needs nurses now more than ever to lead in transformation of our healthcare system, and radically engage in creating justice in health.

3.5   Using Theory of Structuration to Ground Justice in Health

We began our exploration of theory with critical perspectives and their derivatives which include social justice. To attain justice, interrogation of structures is essential given the consequences they generate as a result of their power, oppressive nature, and inequitable practices. Structures are the tangible and intangible components of systems that shape practices (actions and procedures) and influence outcomes. In recent years, acknowledging the role that structures play in influencing health has been elevated in part due to the ever-increasing disparities and the reckoning of race in America. Structures are policies, practices, rules, and resources sanctioned by those with power to organize entities such institutions, organizations, government, and businesses. They range from the economic to the social and political and are embedded with actors, individuals who carry out and animate the structure and its operations. Animation of the structure is insidious, evoking consequences that reify its inherent oppression and power imbalances causing violence and harm to its victims. Of importance are structures situated within the broader societal context replete with ideology, values, and norms which interdiscursively promulgate conditions of that social context. The result is structuration—a theoretical perspective created by Anthony Giddens (1984) deeply rooted in the traditions of critical social theorist Jürgen Habermas.

Structuration occurs when structural properties of a system extend beyond time or space to influence and affect agency, power, and action. It is defined as "conditions governing the continuity or transmutation of structures and therefore the reproduction of social systems" (Giddens, 1984, p. 25). This creates a duality between actors and the system which recursively reproduce social practices and actions that are either enabling or constraining. The importance of structuration is its ponderance of the absence of individual knowledge that actors have of their role in reifying contextualized structural phenomena that perpetuate intended and unintended conditions. Like a feedback loop, the actors relative unknowing of the contextuality of their actions causes its continued re-creation and reification.

Those groups most vulnerable and marginalized in our society in addition to any viewed as deviant from the centered norm of whiteness and acceptable Western culture, values, and traditions perpetually suffer negative structural consequences.

They are more apt to experience the manifestations of structurally created and structurally sustained inequities that inadvertently cause structural violence.

Burnett et al. studies (Burnett, 2012; Burnett et al., 2018) examine the impact of policies on the delivery of shelter services to women who had been exposed to intimate partner violence first in Canada and then in the United States. Both studies were guided by Giddens's Theory of Structuration and critical feminist theory and used critical discourse analysis to examine how structures affect service delivery. Findings reveal the occurrence of structural violence through the implementation of policies that was perpetrated and reified by actors across systems that created unintended consequences for shelters and the families they serve (Burnett et al., 2015, 2016). There was a tension that became evident between how policies were written and its subsequent enactment that caused unintentional harm even though they were well intended. That harm is structural violence.

3.6   Structural Violence

Structural violence is the insidious assaults that structures perpetrate on those who encounter them. It is the ways that structurally induced and structurally perpetuated inequities violate those most susceptible, disproportionately, and inhumanely. Galtung (1969) the originator of this work defines structural violence as violence that is "built into the structure and shows up as unequal power and consequently as un- equal life chances" (Galtung, 1980, p. 171). By nature, structural violence enacts power inequities in resource distribution which manifest consequences with social justice implications. Galtung (1980) assigns traits to structural violence where "exploitation is at its centerpiece," "unequal exchange" occurs, and there is "built in repression" (pp. 293–294). It is viewed as violence built into a structure that socially interacts with systems, ideology, actors, and power, to the detriment of individuals particularly those with less social collateral, influence, and resources. The violence exerted by structures produces consequences which exacerbate and reinforce disparities further impeding progress and human flourishing. Ho (2017) discusses this theory of violence as "the avoidable disparity between the potential ability to fulfill basic needs and their actual fulfillment" (p. 1). Although this form of violence might feel obtuse, its existence and impacts are as Ho (2017) identified avoidable and taken further, preventable.

Obstacles to preventing structural violence are buried within a complex network of systems, policies, and power. Inequities in the distribution of power influence the equitable distribution of resources, in addition to system drivers and policy products which also play a role in producing structural inequalities which constrain personal agency. The constraining of personal agency is the crime scene of structural violence because it interferes with ones' potential and fulfillment (Ho, 2017).

The role of structures in shaping and constraining human potential and opportunity has been well documented and known. Yet attention to structures has been in the background—obnoxiously overshadowed by an accentuated focus on the individual and individual level interventions as the sole source of outcomes, be it positive or negative. This skewed focus has allowed for the continued violent assault of structures on the human condition that sustain disparities and inequities in communities of color and vulnerable populations.

3.6.1   Structural Racism

For decades, Black people in America and around the world have been subjected to structural racism and its dire consequences resulting in increasing health and social disparities and increased prevalence of disease and death higher than any other population group. The summer of 2020 has brought to bear the perpetually deferred reckoning with and candid acknowledgment of racism in America and its deep entrenchment in all structures. When we saw the barbaric killing of George Floyd and many other African Americans, we saw moments of some of the deepest most profound eruption of racism and structural racism witnessed in modern history. We bore witness not only the murder of a human being but also the inhumanity of racism and how it has infiltrated our most esteemed systems and actors within those systems. That reality is forcing the consciousness of our country to cross a threshold of acknowledging racism and its structural permutations. It has shifted our national mood to demand urgent and immediate action steps to eradicate racism in all its forms, including structural racism.

We are experiencing the repercussions of this systemically entrenched racist history and racist practices continue to cause disparity and fracture the very foundations of trust of health disciplines and of science.

Nursing, with its long-standing history of allegiance to social justice values and practice, has also disseminated renewed calls to action, action reports, and position statements as reminders of the profession's moral imperative to address social injustice, inequity, and health disparities. Although none of these issues are new to nursing or medicine, these health professions make up the majority of our healthcare system. What is new, however, are the increasing calls from within and externally to do something in a much more meaningful and actionable way to address issues of inequity and social justice. These "call to action" statements and documents are at best an initial attempt to move beyond acknowledgment of the existence of disparity to outlining recommendations to thwart it. More challenging than articulating and implementing these action calls are embedding them deeply within the profession and the system so that they live beyond a report, a document, or a statement. They must persist beyond a reaction to a moment in time and instead live in perpetuity inherently within the system, as a way of being. That is where the critical chasm of inequity persists—between identifying what is hoped for (aspiration) and what is (reality) which has caused ineffective progress generation after generation. We have been revisiting the same issues and getting the same, if not worse, results and outcomes. Health disparities in the United States are increasing, not decreasing, as are gaps in income, wealth, and opportunity.

The scourge of racism repeatedly rears its ugly head in our society, in our institutions, and yes, even in our own healthcare professions. The issues are predictable and the negative health outcomes known, and yet, we still proceed along ineffective directions to remedy the situation. Justice in health pursues a sustained effort to remedy and rectify the problems at its root with the expectation of achieving a different outcome; an outcome that improves and creates health. So why, thus far, as a collective of highly skilled and knowledgeable health professions has addressing and ameliorating the array of health inequity and social justice issues been seemingly so difficult? A significant part of the answer lies directly on the historical laser focus of our system of care and its professionals on the individual decontextualized from their environment and the factors that undermine their health. Sickness is addressed more readily than prevention is embraced, which is seen by the amount of investment in public health compared to medical institutions. Moreover, there is less emphasis on root causes and the structural scaffolding that upholds the status quo which allows for the active and passive perpetuation of injustice, racism, and inequity.

3.7   Structural Justice

Remedying structural injustice to create justice in health needs the engagement of a new critically informed perspective. Structural justice prioritizes structural attentiveness and structurally driven strategies to generate equitable and just solutions. Recalling our earlier discussion about structures and structuration is foundational to the understanding of structural justice. According to Burnett, Swanberg, Hudson and Schminkey (2018):

> Structural justice acknowledges the oppressive and re-victimizing inherent nature of structures as unacceptable and requires purposeful rectification. It demands that primacy and privilege be extended to the most vulnerable, through sustainable structural processes that attend to equity, power and human dignity.
>
>   It declares the unacceptability of current structural conditions as unjust and violent. Through a structural justice lens, existing structures are viewed as intolerable and disruptive to individual autonomy and impediments to well-being. Importantly, no particular blame is placed on existing entities. Instead, structural justice illuminates the inherent nature of the system and its actors' behaviors to unintentionally and implicitly create injustice and structural violence (p. 62).

The notion of structural justice builds on justice literature by integrating the core elements of various forms of justice most applicable to deepening our understanding of structural inequity. Uniquely, the foundational tenets of structural justice are informed by dialogue from a study examining systemic effects on agencies that provide services to abused women. Although the population might vary, the vulnerability remains the constant thread which allows for adaptability of this approach. Grounding structural justice as a theory will require additional exploration and structured use in study design and implementation to test its resolve. In the meantime, it can still be used as a guiding framework to begin to redress many of the inequities and health injustices facing diverse communities and disparate populations.

Structural justice is the missing link to structural reform not only in health care but also across many of the spaces and systems where health happens. Health happens at home, in schools, and in communities and is enabled or constrained by institutions, policies, and actors. Structural justice addresses that which constrains and enables health wherever it happens using essential tenets to direct and animate its mission.

3.7.1 Tenets of Structural Justice

The tenets of structural justice derive from the critical elements of multiple forms of justice that were amalgamated to inform the evolution of structural justice. These elements, along with distilling the narratives of system actors, were also used in the development of these tenets. It is important to note that system actors can be both witnesses and perpetrators. They can also be "a part of" the system yet "removed from" determining its harmful mechanisms such as insufficient funding appropriations, policy incongruence across external agencies, regulatory mandates, etc. In this case, the narratives came from system actors working within a system that delivers services to abused women nested in a larger systemic web of agencies, policies, and actors which constrain and enable the work they do and how they do it. The sharing of their insider experiences and the impacts they witnessed helped deepen our understanding of structural injustice and inform the imagining of structural justice and its five essential tenets (Burnett, Swanberg, Hudson and Schminkey, 2018).

The five essential tenets of structural justice are:

1. The Critical Acknowledgment of Intersectionality and Oppression.
2. Multidimensional Accessibility and Coordination.
3. Buffering Vulnerability.
4. Intentional Equalization Through Equity.
5. Elevated Consciousness and Action.

It has become increasingly clear that these tenets are crucial to drive the concurrent goals of health equity and health sovereignty which need the actualization of justice in health to be achieved. The ensuing discussion of the structural justice tenets occur through the convergent lens of structural justice and justice in health.

3.7.2 The Critical Acknowledgment of Intersectionality and Oppression

Critical acknowledgment fosters transparency and candor about the facts, void of convenient omissions and baseless alternatives. It makes it unequivocally known that identity has multiple forms and oppression has been a long-standing culprit, each affecting outcomes. To be critical is not to criticize, it is to examine unencumbered the historical and present reality that exists for those most vulnerable, often excluded from the dominant discourse. Such reality must be affirmed by truth telling of inequity and injustices and their consequences seen and unseen. Rooted within a critical orientation, structural justice assumptions are ideologically consistent within that paradigm. Structural justice assumes inequity and injustice that need to be corrected. It assumes diversity and intersectionality of lived experiences and identity. It assumes that structures are inherently powerful and that the power is inequitable in its distribution resulting in oppression of those with the least amount of power or access to power. Acknowledgment of systemic and structural history's role in perpetuating and creating inequity and injustice provides knowledge that can be used to address the intended and unintended consequences of that history. It is an act of recognition that names the problem at its core: a crucial starting point for change. Problem identification should lead first to understanding the history and impact of the problem and secondly, how that impact is experienced by different populations, communities, and individuals shaped by their location and identity. To foster equity and equitable solutions, difference, diversity, and the entwining dynamics of each as precipitating factors for beginning to redress and reconcile the problem must be considered. Fully creating justice in health requires the removal of problematic structural impediments to achieving health sovereignty and rectifying problematic structural deficiencies. Rectifying structural deficiencies occur by creating structures that are inherently just and eliminating those that are not.

We are at the precipice of a historical opportunity to make long overdue structural changes to our system of care. Increasing healthcare costs that are not improving health outcomes relative to what is being spent is a problem. Health outcomes in the United States are diminishing with decreasing mortality rates (Muennig et al., 2018) as cost continue to rise, unsustainably. The United States spends more than any other developed nation in the world attributing to almost 18% of its GDP (Tikkanen & Abrams, 2019; https://www.cms.gov/Research-Statistics-Data-and-Systems/Statistics-Trends-and-Reports/NationalHealthExpendData/NationalHealthAccountsHistorical) with worst outcomes (Tikkanen & Abrams, 2019; Papanicolas et al., 2018).

COVID-19 only exacerbated the system cracks such as impacts to access to care, effects on the quality and affordability of care, and widening health disparities and mortality gaps (Kurani et al., 2020) that already existed. Workforce depletion and supply chain failures indicate a healthcare system in need of a serious reset that cannot be informed by old patterns and practices of the past. This illumination has catapulted the urgency to reform these structures to levels not seen in recent years.

Reforming the current system must incorporate the intentional "building in" of justice in health where structures that create health sustain health and mitigate threats to health. A broad scale systematic examination of many facets within the spectrum of health such as workforce practices, unintended consequences of policies and procedures, the redefining of health, the reimagining of healthcare settings, the diminishing of the dominant health narratives and practices that are harmful, the inclusion of historically excluded voices, and the intention resetting of the health agenda from sick care domination to prevention and public health informed by structural justice. This begins with critical acknowledgment and subsequent deliberate action to redress gaps and deficiencies with new approaches and orientations.

3.7.3   Multidimensional Accessibility and Coordination

Access to care is often at the heart of most health equity efforts. For too long, having a service has been equated with being able to access the service and access it unencumbered. Through the foundational study of shelter service delivery to abused women (Burnett, 2012; Burnett et al., 2015, 2016), shelters often found it challenging to support families in living violence-free lives due to the siloed configuration of the systems that they engaged with and that women needed to access. This presented many navigation issues and coordination struggles amidst a web of unnecessary complexity which created structural violence—another form of abuse that re-victimized an already vulnerable population.

Similar challenges also occur outside of the shelter delivery context. This is an age-old problem in the configuration of systems at large and the lack of congruence between their execution of services, resources, and programs and disconnection between policies, practices, and procedures from one agency to the next. At the center are the clients who at times need the support of many agency partners, simultaneously. Individuals face the daunting task of navigating each point of agency entry where they must learn the rules of that agency and decipher how its policy relates not only to their circumstance but also those of other agencies they are involved with. At multiple entry points, clients are retelling their stories, facing obstacles to services and decisions that can negatively impact their outcomes. The onus for being able to access the system and coordinate services successfully should not fall to the client. It is the responsibility of the system to be designed to interact within itself to the betterment of the client.

Structural justice expects systems to function in alignment, congruence and nimbly in addressing the needs of those it is intended to serve. A system is just in its structures when its policies and practices are implemented in ways and by actors that do not cause unintended consequences, harm, or violence. The "system" intentionally examines and evaluates itself for what is not working and rectifies it so that it can work optimally. Such a system anticipates in its design loop holes and pitfalls that might entangle its users into untenable circumstances and is inherently designed to avoid this at all costs. It listens to and is informed by the users' experiences. It is a system that is solution-driven and sets its clients up for success by infusing intersectionality, antiracism, healing and compassion into its expectations. Such a system will be coordinated and aligned across sectors and disciplines to best respond to the needs of its most vulnerable. It will have done the necessary diligence to ensure that it is coordinated and accessible across populations, communities, and identities in multiple forms.

3.7.4 Buffering Vulnerability

Hidden realities of vulnerable individuals are masked in how systems respond to the obvious and presenting vulnerability be it poverty, homeless, or violence. A system response which buffers vulnerability is one that understands the extent of vulnerability and implements measures that do not reinforce that vulnerability. An example from the case of abused women seeking shelter services, structural justice contends that adding "sensible levels of social protection that are undergirded by principles of trauma and violence informed care" are essential "to promote better overall help seeking experiences; enhance system encounter experiences and minimize harm to women" (Burnett et al., 2018, p. 61). In this situation, the spectrum of vulnerability in this population requires that system supports offer trauma-informed approach principles and approaches at points of contact to safeguard vulnerability. More broad expansion of buffering vulnerability reflects the factoring in of the individuals' hidden realities that are exposed through intentional holistic inquiry of the totality of their lived experiences. It is structures that synergistically address the confounding issues affecting health outcomes and values understanding health through all of the determinants.

A system guided by structural justice acts to resolve impediments to achieving health equitably and creates justice in health when it can identify vulnerability and mobilize its implementation to avoid exacerbating vulnerability or causing additional vulnerability. Buffering happens in the space where complex lives often meet misaligned system approaches that are geared to help people. Often, what occurs in this space is predictable and well known by those who have been caught up in its midst. In the case of the study of agencies that support women exposed to violence, the space that requires buffering is that where policies of no contact orders and custody orders are in conflict and contradict each other; it is the space where women in shelter have 30–45 allowable shelter stay days to reconstruct their lives yet there are no affordable housing options available for them to go to, and even if they are available, the waiting lists are years long.

These examples demonstrate that complex circumstances require solutions that compassionately respond to pressing needs. Having space in shelter for abused women and children are important for them to flee abusive relationships. However, if there are no viable options for abused women when they leave, or they are put in a position where ongoing contact with an abuser is required for visitation, then we have not protected their vulnerability—we have only added to it. Now the women and their children could be homeless, forced to return to the abuser as a result of having nowhere else to go, exposed to further and escalating abuse, and suffer health consequences from that prolonged exposure. We have now created a situation where the risk to the family increases, and their need for additional resources could also increase due to exacerbation of the issues that were not properly buffered in the first place. Having a system that buffers vulnerability means that simply offering services, programs, resources, and support is not enough. It must also contend with how it can sensibly protect and apply itself without causing harm and increasing

vulnerability. Vulnerability disproportionately occurs in populations that are marginalized, racialized, gendered, and impoverished. Because of this, learning how
best to buffer vulnerability must first be applied with knowledge of the critical tipping points for those deemed to be vulnerable and prioritized by restorative action.

3.7.5 Intentional Equalization Through Equity

To be intentional is to engage with purpose toward an end that leads to results reflective of the intended outcome. Structural justice does not assume that intention and
outcomes are aligned when actions, policies, or practices are at work. Instead, it
insists that they are not and therefore concerted efforts have to be made to meet and
keep this alignment. Being well intended does not guarantee optimal outcomes and
structural justices looks beyond the surface of intention to results which is where the
truest manifestation of the consequences of the intention appear. It is at this end of
the spectrum where structural justice inserts itself by illuminating the consequences
and providing the remedy. The remedy proposed by this tenant of structural justice
is to intentionally equalize the consequences so that they are equitable and just.
Using the example again from the shelter services study of abused women, this tenet
focuses on the intentional equalization of the systems' orientation around access
and resources that support abused women and their children as informed by field
experts. It directly responds to findings that point to three key area where such
equalization is warranted: (1) the need for sufficient funding appropriations to such
agencies so they can meet the unique and varied needs of this population; (2)
improved system access to sufficient to meet their client's needs; and (3) sensible
policy implementation across institutions (Burnett, Swanberg, Hudson, and
Schminkey, 2018).

Government funding appropriations, in particular, are term limited and restric-
tive in how they can be used which impedes the amount and type of service and
support that agencies can offer to their clients. The need of the clients and the funding allotment are rarely equivalent nor aligned. Therefore, equalization of funding
appropriations would allow funding to be applied in amounts proportionate to the
scale and extent of the need—determined by content experts. Their wisdom helps
open opportunities for more precise and creative use of funding dollars. It would
give autonomy of agencies to determine how best to spend dollars for maximal
benefit to their services and consumers.

Issues of system access and policy enactment can detrimentally hinder the client's experience in the system and their outcomes. This takes the form of siloed
systems that do not communicate, coordinate, or use cumbersome access processes.
Variable points of access across multiple systems of support leaves policies which
guide and influence service delivery also fractured. Instead, they roll out in isolation
and lack of the ability to empathically respond to unique circumstances or predica-
ments that often require more than a one-size-fits-all approach. Equity matters in all
things at the heart of structures and their functioning which includes funding,

access, and policies. We have to ensure that where structural inequities exist, we intentionally equalize them to alleviate the undue harm, stress, and negative outcomes they create. Otherwise, we perpetuate all that we are trying to mitigate and our efforts to improve health cannot be achieved. Worse, they are futile. Justice in health begins with the intentional formation of structural justice as its platform to establish equitable and just health care.

3.7.6 Elevated Consciousness and Action

Elevating one's consciousness brings the unknown into knowingness. As rudimentary as this sounds, until such awareness occurs it is almost impossible to conceive of the correct course of action let alone informed and conscientious actions. You must come into awareness of knowledge before you can act on it, and that awareness has to originate from "new" knowing. Applying what you know within our repository of knowledge may be insufficient to properly address or conceive of appropriate solutions. Simply, your own perception and perspective are not enough to foster new knowing because the point of reference for your knowledge is limited by the extent of your exposures and experiences. Those exposure and experiences are influenced and shaped by the context of your life which although unique is also similar to people with the same types of experiences and exposures. What is missing are those exposures and experiences that are unlike your own or least like what is familiar to you.

Critical approaches acknowledge that when we show up, we come with our experiences, inherent biases, values, and beliefs as well. These tacitly affect our thinking and our responses. Elevating our consciousness intentionally forces us to become aware of those other experiences and exposures that fall outside of our default and uses those to also fuel our knowledge and insight into a new realm, one that is different from our own. Repeated exposure to difference and diversity, to experiences and stories (unlike one's own), and situations which strike a moral chord are more likely to help elevate consciousness to the spectrum of the human condition and diaspora of lived experiences. However, it has to be actively sought out and reflected upon; otherwise no elevation of consciousness can occur. As consciousness elevates, there is an expectation to assess and act on the knowledge. Assessment of the new knowledge is examination of its substance for inherent fairness, justice, and equity. This should be an iterative process of examination, internal interrogation, evaluation, and action.

Structural justice assumes that identification of fairness, justice, and equity will occur when insight into experiences are compared across groups, and it is found that certain groups suffer disproportionately negative and harmful outcomes from policy or other structural decisions and processes; hence it is an unfair, unjust, and inequitable condition. Action is the expected response to this conclusion. What that action looks like and how it occurs must target rectifying solutions at all levels with intense focus on the structural. Actions need to be consistent and sustained. Health justice is an outcome of structural justice each interconnected and unachievable without the other.

The onus on healthcare providers to engage in a structural justice mindset should be a heavily weighted expectation and a professional charge in all health-related decision-making irrespective of level. Educating healthcare professionals with this orientation requires an immediate shift in how we prepare healthcare providers. We have experienced many times over the ramifications of not truly prioritizing health equity and justice in health. The evidence of its consequences lies in exacerbation of treatable chronic health conditions and the ever-widening health disparities confounded by escalating healthcare costs. Not addressing the root causes of health has left the full context of the patient untreated and worse has set them up for recurring and concurrent health challenges. It is a stretch to purport to be about the business of health yet not attend to known structural conditions and systems that diminish it. As much as the importance of such a perspective could be argued, given the lack of progress in eliminating disparities and injustice, clearly the case still needs to be made. The case is that health is a human right and that as keepers of health, we have affirmed the moral imperative to uphold health. This means attending all aspects of health, not just parts of it.

There has long been a hyper-focus on the physical conditions and drivers of health in education, preparation, and practice of healthcare providers at the expense of the social and structural determinants of health. Similarly, our systems of health care have been set up to service the physical health needs of the individual and families after they become ill more so than the determinants of health preventatively. Although needed, tertiary care cannot be the dominant line of defense and where most of our investments of knowledge, money, and decisions are made. In treating the total health and well-being of people, equal if not greater amounts of attention have to be paid to the other aspects of a person's humanity that promote health and healing. Given this responsibility and ethical expectation, it is urgently fundamental to our practice that we have an elevated consciousness about the multifaceted realities of the human experience to be able to treat it preventatively, proactively, and when all else fails, reactively.

3.8 The Social Determinants of Health

We have talked about the use of a critical orientation as the framing paradigm that informs structural justice and creates justice in health. Nowhere is justice in health most needed than in the pursuit of social determinants of health and the structures that enable it. The social determinants of health are drivers that determine if we live healthy and healthful lives or foster health disparities and inequities. Depending on the source, the list of social determinants may vary; however, commonly agreed upon social determinants of health include education, housing, income, social status, employment, the built environment, access to food and transportation, etc.

At their core, the social determinants of health are known causal factors that differentiate health outcomes such as morbidity and mortality often along lines of identity, gender, race/ethnicity, ability, geography and income across individuals, populations, and aggregate populations. The United States Department of Health and Human Services Healthy People 2030 initiative (U.S. Department of Health and Human Services, Office of Disease Prevention and Health Promotion, n.d.) outline domains of social determinants of health which they identify as having a "major impact on people's health, well-being, and quality of life" (see Fig. 3.1).

Each domain is composed of some examples of the determinants identified earlier. Importantly, Healthy People 2030 acknowledges upstream approaches as key to diminishing health inequity and disparity.

Without question, the social determinants of health stakes are high and consequences dire which further support the rationale for intentional focus and remedying action. We have frameworks, some discussed here, and others discuss elsewhere, to serve as scaffolding for our approaches and guideposts to solutions. Reorienting our healthcare system and the providers comprising that system will require diverse approaches, ideas, and innovation. Traditional structures need to be upended in favor of better outcomes that utilize new and comprehensive approaches laser focused on structures as critical drivers which influence the social determinants of health.

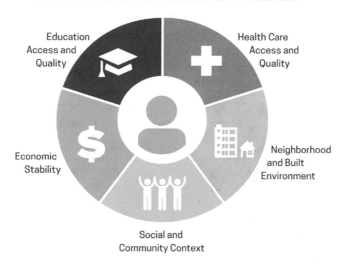

Fig. 3.1 Healthy People 2030 – Social Determinants of Health. (Source: Healthy People 2030, U.S. Department of Health and Human Services, Office of Disease Prevention and Health Promotion, n.d. Retrieved from: https://health.gov/healthypeople/objectives-and-data/social-determinants-health)

3.9   Race as a Determinant of Health

Enacting health and social justice frequently happens from the ground up. It is frequently led by grassroots and not-for-profit organizations that organize around community prioritized issues to make a change locally that ripples nationally. Many locally generated movements such as Black Lives Matter (https://blacklivesmatter. com/) have inspired national agendas and shed a spotlight on issues that disrupt the health of communities and specific populations within communities such as race.

Race is a manufactured construct that shapes the health and health outcomes of Black and Brown people in this country and globally (Jones, 2000). Harrell, 2000 defines race as:

> a system of dominance, power, and privilege based on racial group designations; rooted in the historical oppression of a group defined or perceived by dominant-group members as inferior, deviant, or undesirable; and occurring in circumstances where members of the dominant group create or accept their societal privilege by maintaining structures, ideology, values, and behavior that have the intent or effect of leaving non-dominant-group members relatively excluded from power, esteem, status, and/or equal access to societal resources (Harrell, 2000, p. 43).

Many of the health disparities that exist do so along lines of race and followed closely by geography and zip code which too are often delineated along racial lines as well. Racial health disparities manifest through persistent discrimination, exclusion, and marginalization perpetuated through and embedded within structures, systems, and actors within those systems. The root cause of racial disparities is racism and structural racism is the locality where racist practices are systemically embedded and perpetrated.

Features of structural racism that influence racial health disparities have been consolidated by Hicken et al. (2018) in Box 3.1.

Box 3.1: Features of Structural Racism Important for Racial Health Inequalities

1. Structural racism can be considered the actualization of cultural racism as the latter determines the interdependent formal and informal institutions that comprise the former (Alexander, 2010; Dressler et al., 2005, see "Structural-Constructivist Model").
2. Cultural racism can render the linkages between structural factors and racial health inequalities invisible (Bonilla-Silva, 2010; Fassin, 2004).
3. Structural racism is maintained by multiple, simultaneously acting, and interdependent formal and informal institutions (Powell, 2007).
4. Structural racism is inextricably linked to nation-building and global capitalist markets (Mullings, 2005; Thomas & Clarke, 2013), and these linkages may place economic concerns over human rights concerns making effective intervention challenging (Farmer, 2004; Farmer & Castro, 2004).

(continued)

5. Structural racism includes the erasure of historical processes that could clarify the link between racialized groups and health (Farmer, 2004).
6. As a fundamental cause of racial health inequalities, structural racism continually changes to adapt to contemporary and spatially specific social norms (Mullings, 2005; Silverstein, 2005).
7. Structural racism does not require malicious intent on the part of specific individuals or groups (Harrell, 2000; C. P. Jones, 2000).
8. Structural racism does not require explicit action, as it is often maintained through inaction (Bobo et al., 1997).

(Reprinted from *Social Science & Medicine*, Vol. 199, Hicken, M. T., Kravitz-Wirtz, N., Durkee, M., & Jackson, J. S., *Racial inequalities in health: Framing future research*, p. 11–18, Copyright 2018, with permission from Elsevier.)

3.9.1 Race, Power, and Privilege

Race, power, and privilege, although not frequently named as determinants of health, are proven determinants to accessing and influencing health. It has been established that the United States was founded on racist practices of colonization which embedded the seed of racism which grew through slavery, Jim Crow, and civil rights movement and continues to grow through health and other disparities (income, education, access to care and opportunity, criminal justice), population-specific negative sequelae that is disproportionate (morbidity, mortality, prevalence, incident), and even COVID-19 (Jones, 2000; CDC, 2021). Other scholars have taken a much deeper dive to provide the facts on the chronological linkages of race, racism, and racist practices. The essence here is that racism is a public health issue (CDC, 2021) that intersects with a variety of outcomes and requires justice in health to remedy because it is a determinant of health.

Opportunity, wealth, options, access, and policy are also important and powerful health spaces. Privilege, the unearned benefits and advantages that one group has compared to another, is often predicated upon race, identity, and socioeconomic status. Both power and privilege shape the lives of the groups who suffer from the highest rates of health disparities and prolific inequities. They are reinforced by those occupying power and privilege impacting many of the health and social challenges such as health disparities, oppression, and dehumanization which plague our society. Nixon (2019) masterfully examined privilege though an anti-oppressive lens emphasizing the need for critical allyship to disrupt the "iterative cycle of benefit" caused by privilege. Unchecked privilege, she argues, can lead to "an irrational sense of entitlement, expertise and access" (Nixon, 2019,

p. 5) that creates actions which reinforce this position and further entrench the system of inequity.

Healthcare systems as with other institutions are not exempt from manifestations of power and privilege within their systems, structures, ideology, and practices which are dehumanizing and oppressive. The dynamic created and perpetuated by institutions of power and their power brokers have not served marginalized and racialized populations optimally. Worse, it has caused harm and will continue to cause harm until it is redressed. Actions that occur within these dominant structures of power will not heal or create health for those who need it the most until they are disrupted and reimagined. Building back better cannot be building back the same. Attention paid to up close and deep examination of privilege is a point of departure for adjusting our position and intentionally creating space and opportunity for those who have been marginalized and excluded from accessing power and privilege. There are many and much needed steps in reforming structures toward structural justice and achieving justice in health.

We must be prepared to deconstruct our ideology around health, infusing our healthcare provider preparation and training with social justice, public health, health equity and health justice principles across all rotations and courses. We must teach healthcare providers to be critical allies who work in solidarity with the community to achieve equity and justice. Our education has to be embedded with reflective practice, cultural humility, and social justice advocacy. This will necessitate the aligning of our licensure examinations to reflect the priority of equity and justice. A commitment to prevention as the default versus sick care would reward and incentivize healthcare providers for fostering healthful environments and radically invest efforts and strategies in health in all policies and practices.

3.10   Conclusion

Justice in Health is the reset that healthcare professionals, health systems, and health consumers need. It enables human flourishing through a just and equitable health system and especially structures and practices that are co-created within communities by those communities. We have seen time and time again that our altruistic belief in the right to health, aspirational statements about health care for all, and individual siloed approaches to treating disease is not enough. We have not tangibly moved the needle in health disparities and health inequities for decades. We began this chapter by laying the foundation of critical approaches as instruments to examine and call out the reality faced by racialized and marginalized populations. Acknowledging systems as unjust, laden with the inequitable distribution of power, and oppressive to many is the starting point of truth from which reconciliation and rectification will occur. This platform of truth is foundational to resetting what is not working and necessary to purposefully achieve the goals that advance Justice in Health. Advancing justice in health is a leveler that facilitates health equity and diminishes the disparities that we purport to care about. It is the act of caring required to take action. It is the act of caring that is a part of and not separate from oaths, commitments, and moral imperatives to do no harm and protect health. From this perspective, justice is not and cannot ever be a one-time affair. It has to be created at every intersection, with every intervention, decision point, and thought. Teaching healthcare providers to be incubators of justice in thought and deed is transformative. The transformation spurred on by such an approach invokes a deep level of reflection that transforms our practices, our policies, and our structures.

Justice in health is clarifying solutions that prioritize not only the client's needs but also their strengths and expertise. It is inclusive of innovative thought, is transdisciplinary, and targets sustained and equitable action particularly across systems, health determinants, and structures.

3.11   Reflective Questions and Considerations

1. Ask yourself how the work you are doing is transformative and whom is it transformative for?
2. Who is benefiting the most and are you co-creating health by attending to root causes and including the voices of those who need it the most?
3. Justice in health takes intentional work, intentional change, and intentional action. So what is your intention and does the manifestation of that intention match your actions?

References

Alexander, M. (2010). *The new jim crow: Mass incarceration in the age of colorblindness*.

Baptiste, D. L., Turner, S., Josiah, N., Arscott, J., Alvarez, C., Turkson-Ocran, R. A., et al. (2021). Hidden figures of nursing: The historical contributions of black nurses and a narrative for those who are unnamed, undocumented and underrepresented. *Journal of Advanced Nursing, 77*(4), 1627–1632.

Bobo, L., Kluegel, J. R., Smith, R. A. (1997). Laissez-faire racism: The crystallization of a kinder, gentler, antiblack ideology. In: Tuch SA, Martin JK (Eds.), *Racial attitudes in the 1990s: Continuity and change* (pp. 15–42). Westport, CT: Praeger.

Bohman, J. (2005). *Critical theory. Stanford Encyclopedia of Philosophy*. Retrieved June 17, 2022, from https://plato.stanford.edu/entries/critical-theory/?utm_source=mandiner&utm_medium=link&utm_campaign=mandiner_202108

Bonilla-Silva, E. (2010). *Racism without racists: Color-blind racism and the persistence of racial inequality in America*. Lanham, MD: Rowman & Littlefield.

Brown, K., & Jackson, D. D. (2013). The history and conceptual elements of critical race theory. In *Handbook of critical race theory in education* (pp. 29–42). Routledge.

Buhler-Wilkerson, K. (1993). Bringing care to the people: Lillian Wald's legacy to public health nursing. *American Journal of Public Health, 83*(12), 1778–1786.

Burnett, C. (2012). *Examining the effects of policies on the delivery of shelter services to women who have experienced intimate partner violence*. Dissertation. University of Western Ontario Libraries.

Burnett, C., Ford-Gilboe, M., Berman, H., Ward-Griffin, C., & Wathen, N. (2015). A critical analysis of provincial policies impacting shelter service delivery to women exposed to violence. *Politics, Policy and Nursing Journal, 16*(1–2), 5–16. https://doi.org/10.1177/1527154415583123

Burnett, C., Ford-Gilboe, M., Berman, H., Wathen, N., & Ward-Griffin, C. (2016). Day to day reality of shelter service delivery to abused women in the context of system and policy demands. *Journal of Social Service Research*. https://doi.org/10.1177/1527154415583123

Burnett, C., Swanberg, M., Hudson, A., & Schminkey, D. (2018, Winter). Structural justice: A critical feminist framework exploring the intersection between justice, equity and structural reconciliation. *Journal of Health Disparities Research and Practice, 11*(4), 52–68.

Centers for Disease Control and Prevention. (2021). Retrieved from June 21, 2021, from https://www.cdc.gov/healthequity/racism-disparities/index.html

Centers for Disease Control and Prevention. *Cases of coronavirus disease (COVID-19) in the U.S.* Retrieved from: www.cdc.gov/coronavirus/2019-ncov/cases-updates/cases-in-us.html on 20 April 2020.

Centers for Disease Control and Prevention. Provisional death counts for coronavirus disease (COVID-19): Weekly state-specific data updates by select demographic and geographic characteristics. Retrieved from: www.cdc.gov/nchs/nvss/vsrr/covid_weekly on 20 April 2020.

Corradetti, C. (2012). *The Frankfurt School and critical theory. The internet encyclopedia of philosophy.* Retrieved May 16, 2022, from https://art.torvergata.it/retrieve/handle/2108/176490/350218/The%20Frankfurt%20School%20Internet%20Encyclopedia%20of%20Philosophy.pdf

Crenshaw, K. (1991, July). Mapping the margins: Intersectionality, identity politics, and violence against women of color. *Stanford Law Review, 43*(6), 1241–1299.

Crenshaw, K. W. (2010). Twenty years of critical race theory: Looking back to move forward. *Connecticut Law Review, 43*, 1253.

Crewe, S. (2007). Harriet Tubman's last work. *Journal of Gerontological Social Work, 49*(3), 229–244. https://doi.org/10.1300/J083v49n03_13

Critical and Creative Thinking. (2007). Vol 15 (1).

Devetak, R. (2005). Critical theory. *Theories of International Relations, 3*, 137–160.

Donohoe, M., & Schiff, G. (2014). A call to service: Social justice is a public health issue. *Virtual Mentor, 16*(9), 699–707. https://doi.org/10.1001/virtualmentor.2014.16.9.ecas2-1409

Dressler, W. W., Oths, K. S., Gravlee, C. C. (2005) Race and ethnicity in public health research: Models to explain health disparities. *Annual Review of Anthropology, 34*, 231–252.

Falk-Rafael, A. (2005). Speaking truth to power: Nursing's legacy and moral imperative. *Advances in Nursing Science, 28*(3), 212–223.

Farmer, P., & Sidney, W. (2004). Mintz lecture for 2001 - An anthropology of structural violence. *Current Anthropology, 45*, 305–325.

Farmer, P., & Castro, A. (2004). Pearls of the Antilles? Public health in Haiti and Cuba. In: Castro A, Singer M (Eds.), *Unhealthy health policy: a critical anthropological examination* (pp. 3–28). Walnut Creek, Calif: AltaMira Press.

Fassin, D. (2004). Social illegitimacy as the foundation of health inequality: How the politcal treatment of immigrants illuminates a French paradox. In: Castro A, Singer M (Eds.), *Unhealthy health policy: a critical anthropological examination* (pp 203–214). Walnut Creek, Calif: AltaMira Press.

Galtung, J. (1969). Violence, peace and peace research. *Journal of Peace Research, 6*(3), 167–191.

Galtung, J. (1980). Cultural violence. *Journal of Peace Research, 27*(3), 291–307.

Giddens, A. (1984). *The constitution society: The outline of theory of structuration*. University of California Press.

Grande, D., Asch, D. A., & Armstrong, K. (2007). Do doctors vote? *Journal of General Internal Medicine, 22*(5), 585–589.

Gruen, R. L., Campbell, E. G., & Blumenthal, D. (2006). Public roles of US physicians: Community participation, political involvement, and collective advocacy. *Journal of the American Medical Association, 296*(20), 2467–2475.

Harrell, S. P. (2000) A multidimensional conceptualization of racism-related stress: Implications for the well-being of people of color. *American Journal of Orthopsychiatry, 70*, 42–57.

Healthy People 2030, U.S. Department of Health and Human Services, Office of Disease Prevention and Health Promotion. (n.d.). *Social determinants of health.* Retrieved July 22, 2021, from https://health.gov/healthypeople/objectives-and-data/social-determinants-health

Hicken, M. T., Kravitz-Wirtz, N., Durkee, M., & Jackson, J. S. (2018). Racial inequalities in health: Framing future research. *Social Science & Medicine, 1982*(199), 11–18. https://doi.org/10.1016/j.socscimed.2017.12.027

Ho, K. (2017, September). Structural violence as a human rights violation. *Essex Human Rights Review, 4*(2), 1–17.

Horkheimer, M. (1972). *"The social function of philosophy" in critical theory: Selected essays.* New York: Herder and Herder.

Hoggan, C., Mälkki, K., & Finnegan, F. (2017). Developing the theory of perspective transformation: Continuity, intersubjectivity, and emancipatory praxis. *Adult Education Quarterly, 67*(1), 48–64.

Jones, C. P. (2000). Levels of racism: A theoretic framework and a gardener's tale. *American Journal of Public Health, 90*, 1212–1215.

Kurani, N., Kamal, R., Twitter, K. A., Ramirez, G, & Twitter, C.C., (2020). *State of the U.S. Health System: 2020 update.* Kaiser Family Foundation. Retrieved August 9, 2021, from https://www.healthsystemtracker.org/brief/state-of-the-u-s-health-system-2020-update/

Lutz, K., Jones, Dupree, K., & Kendall, J. (1997, December). Expanding the praxis debate: Contributions to clinical inquiry. *Advances in Nursing Science, 20*(2), 23–31.

McLaughlin, N. (1999). Origin myths in the social sciences: Fromm, the Frankfurt School and the emergence of critical theory. *Canadian Journal of Sociology/Cahiers canadiens de sociologie*, 109–139.

Muennig, P., Reynolds, M., Fink, D., Zafari, Z., & Geronimus, A. (2018, December). America's declining Well-being, health, and life expectancy: Not just a white problem. *American Journal of Public Health, 108*(12), 1626–1631. https://doi.org/10.2105/AJPH.2018.304585

Mullings, L. (2005). Interrogating racism: Toward an antiracist anthropology. *Annual Review of Anthropology, 34*, 667–693.

National Geographic. (2013). *Mary Secole.* Retrieved May 14, 2022, from https://www.national-geographic.org/article/mary-seacole/

Nixon, S. (2019). The coin model of privilege and critical allyship: Implications for health. *BMC Public Health, 19*, 1637. https://doi.org/10.1186/s12889-019-7884-9

Papanicolas, I., Woskie, L. R., & Jha, A. K. (2018). Health care spending in the United States and other high-income countries. *Journal of the American Medical Association, 319*(10), 1024–1039. https://doi.org/10.1001/jama.2018.1150

Parsons, J., & Harding, K. (2011). Post-colonial theory and action research. *Turkish Online Journal of Qualitative Inquiry, 2*(2), 1–6.

Patel, N. (2015). Health and social justice: The role of Today's physician. *AMA Journal of Ethics, 17*(10), 894–896. https://doi.org/10.1001/journalofethics.2015.17.10.fred1-1510

Patten, N. A. (1986). The nineteenth century black woman as social reformer: The "new" speeches of sojourner truth. *Negro History Bulletin, 49*(1), 2–5.

Patton, M. (2002). *Qualitative research and evaluation methods* (3rd ed.). Sage.

Peek, M. E., Wilson, S. C., Bussey-Jones, J., et al. (2012). A study of national physician organizations' efforts to reduce racial and ethnic disparities in the United States. *Academic Medicine, 87*(6), 694–700.

Peter A. M., Megan, R., David S. F., Zafar Z., & Arline T. G. (2018). ScD America's declining well-being, health, and life expectancy: Not just a white problem. *American Journal of Public Health, December, 108*(12), 1626–1631. https://doi.org/10.2105/AJPH.2018.304585

Philips, D. (1999). Healthy heroines: Sue Barton, Lillian Wald, Lavinia Lloyd Dock and the Henry Street Settlement. *Journal of American Studies, 33*(1), 65–82.

Powell, J. A. (2007). Structural racism: Building upon the insights of John Calmore. *NCL Review, 86*, 791.

Rukundwa, L. S., & Van Aarde, A. G. (2007). The formation of postcolonial theory. *HTS Teologiese Studies/Theological Studies, 63*(3), 1171–1194.

Sellman, D. (2005). Towards an understanding of nursing as a response to human vulnerability. *Nursing Philosophy, 6*(1), 2–10.

Silverstein, P. A. (2005). Immigrant racialization and the new savage slot: Race, migration, and immigration in the new Europe. *Annual Review of Anthropology, 34*, 363–384.

Staring-Derks, C., Stari, N. J., & Anionwu, E. N. (2015). Mary Seacole: Global nurse extraordinaire. *Journal of Advanced Nursing, 71*(3), 514–525. https://doi.org/10.1111/jan.12559

The Future of Nursing. *2020-2030: Charting a path to achieve health equity*. Retrieved July 13, 2021, from https://www.nationalacademies.org/event/05-11-2021/the-future-of-nursing-2020-2030-charting-a-path-to-achieve-health-equity-report-release-webinar

Thomas, D. A., Clarke, M. K. (2013). Globalization and race: Structures of inequality, new sovereignties, and citizenship in a neoliberal era. *Annual Review of Anthropology, 42*, 305–325.

Tikkanen, R., & Abrams, M. (2019). *U.S. Health Care from a global perspective, higher spending, worse outcomes?* (Commonwealth Fund, Jan. 2020). https://doi.org/10.26099/7avy-fc29. Retrieved from: https://www.commonwealthfund.org/publications/issue-briefs/2020/jan/us-health-care-global-perspective-2019

Tobbell, D., & D'Antonio P. (2022). *The history of racism in nursing: A review of existing scholarship*. Silver Spring, MD: National Commission to Address Racism in Nursing.

United States Government. Centers for Medicare and Medicaid Services. Retrieved August 9, from https://www.cms.gov/Research-Statistics-Data-and-Systems/Statistics-Trends-and-Reports/NationalHealthExpendData/NationalHealthAccountsHistorical.

United States Government. The White House (2021). *American rescue plan: President Biden's plan to provide direct relief to Americans, contain Covid-19, and rescue the economy*. Retrieved May 16, 2022, from https://www.whitehouse.gov/american-rescue-plan/

United States Government: The United States Department of Health and Human Services. (2021). *Healthy people 2030*. Retrieved July 22, 2021, from: https://health.gov/healthypeople/objectives-and-data/social-determinants-health

UVA Today. (2013, January 30). *Nursing forum explores what Nancy Milio's Detroit mom and Tots Clinic did so well*. Retrieved May 14, 2022, from: https://news.virginia.edu/content/nursing-forum-explores-what-nancy-milio-s-detroit-mom-and-tots-clinic-did-so-well

Wikipedia. (2022a). *Florence Nightingale*. Retrieved May 16, 2022, from https://en.wikipedia.org/wiki/Florence_Nightingale

Wikipedia. (2022b). *Mary Secole*. Retrieved May 14, 2022, from https://en.wikipedia.org/wiki/Mary_Seacole

Wolgemuth, J. R., & Donohue, R. (2006). Toward an inquiry of discomfort: Guiding transformation in "emancipatory" narrative research. *Qualitative Inquiry, 12*(5), 1012–1021.

Chapter 4
Health Equity and Critical Health Issues

This chapter dives into exposing critical root causes that perpetuate health dispari-ties such as race, poverty, mass and youth incarceration, and violence against women, communities, and society. It also examines issues that determine health such as access to care, food, housing, transportation, and insurance using concrete examples. Beyond identification of these issues, this chapter makes the connection to earlier perspectives discussed in Chap. 3 to extend and situate health in relation to structural drivers and causes. It is connecting the dots beyond the current health-care orientation that leads to a deepening of understanding of how health happens across disparate populations and in aggregate populations. It also begins to frame what a health equity systems approach could look like and what must be considered.

The health of our nation has been at the foreground of many initiatives spanning generations. Yet we remain struck by and stuck in the ever-present predictable cycle of health disparities, inequities, and injustice. Many of the most pervasive health issues we see, particularly chronic disease and injury, are situational and context-laden while our treatments remain individually targeted. Although necessary, target-ing health solutions at the individual negates the circumstances that continue to cause these very same issues and their re-occurrence. Further the onus for health lies squarely and incorrectly on the individual de-contextualized from their environ-ment. If only Tonya would just eat better or lose weight, her diabetes would get better under control. Why is Donell so non-compliant in taking his medication—he must not want to get that blood pressure under control. From here, treatment ensues to address the disease of diabetes (modification of medication perhaps) and not the condition (external contributing factors like access to healthy food, unemployment). So for Donell and Tonya, another prescription with a stern lecture on the importance of taking medication and adherence to a regiment is expected. What hasn't been addressed?

Story of Tonya

Tonya is a mother of three young children between the ages of 9 and 12 years. She works two jobs while her spouse is employed as an over the road truck driver. His job requires him to be gone for 2-week stints at a time, return home for 3 days, and then back out to repeat the cycle. His employment barely keeps the family afloat; however there are not any other local job opportunities that come close to paying what he's making and that also offers benefits. Tonya has had to take on additional work to help support the family by combining two lower wages jobs just to help cover other family essentials and some of the household bills.

With her husband away most days, and gone for extended periods of time, Tonya juggles most of the household and parenting responsibilities while working long days. She has a 40-min commute to town since they live out on a small acreage in the county where housing is much cheaper and where her husband can park his truck on the days he is home. With 16-h workdays, 6 days per week, there is little time for anything else like preparing home-made meals, exercising, or simply just to rest. Her high stress life is both taxing and draining so much so that when she does have her 1 day off per week, it is spent doing all the things she cannot get done during the week. That time is dominated by chores like laundry, cleaning the house, grocery shopping in town, and trying to spend some time with the children who are often alone during the week.

Attending any routine follow-up healthcare visits are near impossible and very costly, since they require taking unpaid time off work to go to any appointment, not to mention extra gas. So, Tonya saves her limited days for healthcare appointments that are only absolutely necessary for her children. Rest is a luxury as is self-care. Getting a COVID shot or going to the dentist is the least on her list of priorities. Does Tonya know she is diabetic? Yes. Does Tonya want to follow the plan, absolutely.

Although Tonya is being treated for diabetes, what other health issues need attending to that influence her chronic condition? Where is the disconnect here?

Story of Donell
Donell has been struggling to stabilize his hypertension for years. He is in his late 40s and has worked for 25 years, 12-h shifts at the same factory since he was 18 years old in Smallsville, United States, pop. 3600. Although there had been rumors for years of a factory shutdown, Donell was not too worried about it because it seemed so unlikely—until it happened 6 weeks ago. Many of the now unemployed factory workers meet at the main street café trying to figure out what to do next and worrying together about their futures. The payout from the factory was minimal and health benefits only lasted for 30 days. Some people are foregoing trying to secure any additional coverage to save money, while others are scrambling to decide if they should sign up for coverage using the exchange. The payout was just enough to be disqualified for Medicaid and keeping a roof overhead and getting any type of affordable food on the table is the only concern now anyways; the rest will have to wait.

Donell is heading to see his primary care provider to see why he has been having so many headaches lately. It's a visit he is not looking forward to for many reasons and he is uncertain when/if he will be able to see his healthcare provider again. His primary care provider is exasperated with what she perceives as Donell's non-compliant behavior and has sternly expressed her dissatisfaction with his seemingly predictable lack of adherence to her treatment plan. Does Donell know he is hypertensive? Yes. Does he want to follow the plan? Absolutely!

Although Donell is being treated for hypertension, what other health issues need attending to that influence his chronic condition? Where is the disconnect here?

These stories reflect the intersection of health issues that are confounded by the determinants of health. Some are obvious disease culprits, mainly chronic disease, while others are less visible, yet significant influencers of health. While we proceed with examining this critical interface of healthy equity and critical health issues, consider what is not known that should be unearthed to optimize the health and well-being of Tonya and Donell.

4.1   Connecting the Dots: Highlighting Issues at the Praxis of Health and Justice

Health outcomes of disparate populations (poor, Black, Indigenous, Latin x/a/e, people of color, and rural populations) are inextricably shaped by the determinants of health, which are known to cause higher incident rates of disease, disability, and death. Socioeconomic conditions affect healthcare coverage, education, access to healthy food, safe housing, and transportation (Singh et al., 2020). There are so many health influencers including health literacy and digitial equity which shapes how you manage and navigate your health while life expectancy is determined by where you live. Poorer neighborhoods are under-resourced and produce concentrated disadvantage that affect health and well-being (Do et al., 2019; Pinchevsky & Wright, 2012), rates of violence (Pinchevsky & Wright, 2012), and environmental hazards (Banzhaf et al., 2019). Race, ethnicity, gender, and sexual orientation intersect with the determinants of health, further confounding them and diminishing health outcomes to levels that cause marked health disparities across communities and populations.

To simplify the connections, consider individuals/families with lower incomes. Income level will affect where you live, the type of home you live in, the types of foods you are able to buy, the availability of transportation, ability to be insured (fully), if you have internet access and the quality of education. Affordable housing options for low-income families are frequently in neighborhoods of concentrated poverty with limited green space, environmental hazards, underperforming schools, and located in a food and pharmacy deserts with low walkability scores. Personal transportation options are tenuous due to the inability to purchase a new vehicle or maintain the old vehicle. Reliance on public transportation creates longer workdays, unpredictability, and limits options for entertainment, shopping, and appointments. Distribution of income and wealth are inequitable and delineated along racial, gender, and geographical lines. Your identity and conditions predispose you to preventable negative health sequelae.

Rudimentary issues of inequity are pervasive and remain unresolved when unaddressed and/or under addressed at the core. Defining health within the context of justice to ultimately lead to human flourishing and sovereignty illuminates critical and urgent issues that halt progress. In the United States and elsewhere, long-standing issues of race, poverty, opportunity, and disparity impede human progress. Frequently, these are issues experienced in relation to each other, be it directly or indirectly, and co-occur disproportionately across and within groups. Our approaches must match the complexity of health needs by involving multifaceted approaches that better serve the dynamic ecological context of the individual. The individual's health ecosystem requires justice in health to buffer the confounding conditions that prevent health and human flourishing.

The most basic levels of our system of health have not been constructed within equity or justice frameworks, making efforts to truly address health from the place of equity and justice less likely. Instead, we have exceeded our proficiency to treat diseases with a laser focus on biological remedies and providing care for diseases of the body. Poverty, racism, and discrimination are diseases of the human condition, of society, and of communities that drive health of the individual, families, and communities. Herein lies the disconnect between the traditional approaches to health and the remediation abilities of the existing mechanisms to truly achieve health—which lies beyond the absence of physical disease.

Increasingly community grassroots organizations, foundations, and associations have been leading the way in not only amplifying disparities at the intersection of health and justice but are implementing community-based solutions designed to address root causes. Had we risen to meet this challenge with sufficient resources and infrastructure, grassroots mobilization efforts might not have been compelled to lead in this space. While it is expected that cross sector and transdisciplinary collaboration will always be required to mobilize change to do health justice work, the entire system of care has a central role and responsibility in all health spaces. Unfortunately, the lack of an overarching public and population health action agenda has pulled the current system in an unbalanced focus, resulting in organizations and agencies taking stewardship to make health equity and justice in health a reality in a patchwork approach. Later we will showcase some community initiatives as examples of possible solutions to the pervasive issues of health disparities and disparate outcomes for the most vulnerable of populations.

4.2 Violence

Violence occurs in many abusive forms and is perpetuated by people, communities, systems, and structures. Although the consequences of violence may vary, the brunt of impacts are pervasively experienced by marginalized and racialized populations and under-resourced communities. The impact of violence is trauma, and for those who experience multiple forms of violence and/or witness acts of violence, that trauma becomes cumulative and vicarious. Of particular concern is the impact it has on younger generations in creating adverse childhood exposure which lead to negative health outcomes into adulthood. For communities with higher rates of violence, the impacts are seen in PTSD, depression, anxiety impacting overall mental and physcial health.

4.2.1 Gun Violence

We are faced with an epidemic of violence in America most notably gun violence. Over the past several years, gun violence has increased tremendously (see Fig. 4.1). According to the Gun Violence Archive, a not-for-profit organization which has tracked gun violence in the US since 2013, thus far in 2022 (between Jan and August 22, 2022), there have been 428 mass shootings and in excess of 28,000 fatalities attributed to gun violence (https://www.gunviolencearchive.org/). Although this violence is widespread and spans all acts of intention and unintentional gun violence, its effects disproportionately impact Black, Brown, and poor communities.

The Centers for Disease Control and Prevention's (CDC) morbidity and mortality weekly report (Kegler et al., 2022) notes that "with substantial inequities by race and ethnicity and poverty level" (p. 656). This report found "from 2019 to 2020, the overall firearm homicide rate increased 34.6%, from 4.6 to 6.1 per 100,000 persons. The largest increases occurred among non-Hispanic Black or African American males aged 10–44 years and non-Hispanic American Indian or Alaska Native (AI/AN) males aged 25–44 years. Rates of firearm homicide were lowest and increased least at the lowest poverty level and were higher and showed larger increases at higher poverty levels" (Kegler et al., 2022, p. 656).

Eliminating violence requires the intentional dismantling of its strongholds and the disruption of its perpetuating mechanisms. Leading the way in such efforts are community programs and organizations that tackle this issue from different angles. For example, several municipalities have implemented community youth violence prevention programs. National models focus on community-level violence

GVA - *Seven Year Review*	2014	2015	2016	2017	2018	2019	2020
Deaths - Willful, Malicious, Accidental	12,418	13,537	15,112	15,679	14,896	15,448	19,411
Suicides by Gun	21,386	22,018	22,938	23,854	24,432	23,941	Pending
Injuries - Willful, Malicious, Accidental	22,779	27,033	30,666	31,265	28,284	30,186	39,492
Children [aged 0-11] Killed or Injured	603	695	671	733	664	695	999
Teens [aged 12-17] Killed or Injured	2,318	2,695	3,140	3,256	2882	3,122	4,142
Mass Shooting	269	335	382	346	336	417	611
Murder-Suicide	624	530	549	608	623	632	573
Defensive Use [DGU]	1,531	1,393	2,001	2,107	1874	1,597	1,478
Unintentional Shooting	1,605	1,969	2,202	2,039	1691	1,905	2,315

Number of Deaths, Injuries, Children, Teens killed/injured [actual numbers]
Mass Shooting, Murder-suicides, Defensive Use, Unintentional Shooting [number of incidents]
Suicide numbers supplied by CDC End of Year Report [actual numbers]

@gundeaths
www.gunviolencearchive.org
www.facebook.com/gunviolencearchive   ©2021 - GUN VIOLENCE ARCHIVE   GVA

Fig. 4.1 Gun Violence Archive 7-year review. (Source: Gun Violence Archive 2021. Research Data by Gun Violence Archive. Reprinted with permission. Retrieved from https://www.gunviolencearchive.org/)

intervention and prevention such as CURE violence (cvg.org) which uses a disease and behavior framework to impact their ultimate goal of creating a world without violence. Another community violence prevention group are violence interrupters (https://www.violenceinterrupters.org/) who work primarily with street-level gangs to stop retaliation and bring non-violent conflict resolution.

Given the scope and scale of this public health emergency, targeted implementation of multiple strategies is required to deal with the issue of ongoing violence, at-risk populations, and prevention. The CDC (2022) has created a technical package with proposed evidence-based strategies, approaches, and examples of programs, policies, and practices that address violence risk and prevention. These strategies and approaches include:

(a) Strengthening Economic Supports: *Individual and household financial security.*
(b) Promote Family Environments that Support Healthy Development: *Early childhood home visitation/Parenting skill and family relationships programs.*
(c) Provide Quality Education Early in Life: *Preschool enrichment with family engagement.*
(d) Strengthen Young People's Skills: *Universal school-based programs/Job training and employment programs (new).*
(e) Connect Youth to Caring Adults and Activities: *Mentoring Programs/Afterschool programs.*
(f) Create Protective Environments: *Modify the physical and social environment; Reduce exposure to community-level risks; Street outreach and community norm change; Improve school climate and safety.*
(g) Intervene to Lessen Harms and Prevent Future Risk: *Treatment to lessen harms of violence exposure, Treatment to prevent problem behavior and future involvement in violence, Hospital-community partnerships* (CDC, 2022, https://www.cdc.gov/violenceprevention/communityviolence/prevention.html).

Advocacy organizations such as Black Lives Matter (https://blacklivesmatter.com/), Mothers Against Drunk Driving (https://www.madd.org/), March for Our Lives (https://marchforourlives.com/), and Moms Demand Action (https://momsdemandaction.org/) have mobilized movements and policy change around specific acts of violence. Family violence intervention efforts have been shepherded through legislation such as the Violence Against Women Act (https://www.govtrack.us/congress/bills/117/s3623), domestic violence helplines, and associations to end violence against women (National Coalition Against Domestic Violence (NCADV); National Network to End Domestic Violence (NNEDV)).

Interpersonal Violence

Violence happens in the home, a phenomenon known as domestic violence or intimate partner violence is experienced by one in four women in the United States (https://ncadv.org/statistics; CDC, 2021a, b, c, d, e) and globally. It is rooted in power and control and affects the physical (pain, headaches, gastrointestinal disorders, traumatic brain injury) and psychological health (depression, anxiety, PTSD) of those who experience it (CDC, 2021a, b, c, d, e). The consequences of intimate partner violence are far reaching and can even lead to death, strangulation, and suicide. When women leave an intimate partner, many must seek shelter for themselves and their children meaning choosing homelessness. Often those going to shelter already have limited resources or limited access to resources and already face multiple vulnerabilities (immigrant status, poverty, lack of social support, lower socioeconomic status). While in shelter, women are tasked with rebuilding their lives in unrealistic time frames and overcoming a myriad of policies that affect their ability to live violence free (Burnett et al., 2015). Policies of child custody, orders of protection, public housing, child welfare, and public assistance intersect and challenge how women are able to move through their circumstances (Burnett et al., 2016). Each of these points of access has requirements and procedures that inadvertently create negative consequences for families. Furthermore, access to healthy food, housing, ability to secure living wages, transportation, and childcare can easily thwart options for women and their children. What might seem easy such as putting down security deposits for a new apartment or getting an electric bill in your name can be near impossible for the abused.

4.3 Structural Violence as Racism

What happens when the perpetrator of violence is not an individual but a system? It is structural violence—violence that is insidiously exerted by systems actors through systemic structures of unjust policies and procedures with disproportionate consequences to the most marginalized populations.

Structural racism occurs when structural violence is overrepresented along racial lines. Remedying this injustice from a health justice perspective is the infusion of the principles of structural justice. Structural justice intently focuses on areas where structural injustice occurs within systems to rectify and create justice within that system. The creation of systemic justice encourages the configuration of just systems at the onset and in cases where that has not occurred, it provides the principles to make it happen (Burnett, Swanberg, Hudson and Schminkey, 2018). One of the most poignant examples of the intersection of structural violence and structural racism is in the criminal justice system. *The Huffington Post* published a shocking blog in 2016 outlining 18 different areas where racism shows up in the criminal legal system (https://www.huffpost.com/entry/18-examples-of-racism-in-criminal-legal-system_b_57f26bf0e4b095bd896a1476). Black and Brown people are more likely to be stopped by the police, arrested, convicted, and sentenced to lengthy prison terms than whites even "after accounting for relevant legal differences such as crime severity and criminal history" (Ghandnoosh, 2015, p. 11). It is the space where the equal justice initiative has invested its resources and efforts to remediate and rectify inequities and injustice.

4.3.1   Community Exemplar: The Equal Justice Initiative

Equal Justice Initiative is an initiative (https://eji.org/about/) that tackles the violent history and discriminatory practices that disproportionally perpetrated against Black and Brown communities through its focus on criminal justice reform, racial justice, and truth telling education. EJI leans into the assumption of the historically constructed guilt of racialized people, underscoring the critical linkages of poverty, race, and the right to human dignity. They align their efforts to focus on priorities that reflect the areas of disparate burden faced by Black and Brown people and where EJI works intensively to reform, redress, and ameliorate. EJI global priorities encompass key domains of oppression, inequity, and injustice through three crucial goal areas: criminal justice reform, racial justice, and education (See Table 4.1). Within each of these domains are specific elements where targeted efforts are focused for greatest impact.

Overwhelming evidence substantiates the need for an acute attention to justice at large and criminal justice reform more specifically. EJI offers powerful data points which are used to inform the direction of these efforts. Further examination of each of these priorities point to causes of negative health sequelae that in turn produce disparate health outcomes.

Consider just one of these priorities, such as children in adult prison, and its connection to adverse childhood exposure which subsequently lead to an array of negative health outcomes and increased health risk.

According to the US Centers for Disease Control and Prevention (2019), adverse childhood experiences (ACEs) are traumatic events that affect the development of children and are linked to mental health, chronic disease, and substance use issues in adulthood (Adverse Childhood Experiences (ACEs) | VitalSigns | CDC). ACEs affect one in six adults and women and racial/ethnic minorities at higher rates (CDC, 2019). For perspective EJI reports that on any given day in America, 4500 children are housed in adult jail, that 13 states do not have minimum age requirements for prosecuting children as adults, and that children in adult prisons are at greater risk for sexual assault and 9X more likely to commit suicide (Children in Adult Prison (eji.org). Perhaps the issue of children in adult prison might seem to some a "legal" issue. While that fact is not in dispute, a justice in health lens would recognize that children in adult prison cannot be relegated exclusively as a legal issue because it is not. It is a health issue given its ability to cause ACEs among other negative health

Table 4.1   Equal justice initiative priority goals

Criminal justice reform	Racial justice	Education
Death penalty	Legacy of slavery	Just mercy
Children in adult prison	Racial terror	True justice documentary
Wrongful conviction	Lynching	A history of racial injustice calendar
Excessive punishment	Racial segregation	Reports
Prison conditions	Presumption of guilt	Videos
	Community remembrance project	

outcomes which manifest into serious adult health issues. Those adult issues present themselves in every primary healthcare office, emergency department, and surgical units across the country, and our response to these presentations cannot be to simply manage the presenting issue, but to uproot the underlying condition.

4.4   The Social Determinants and Drivers of Health

The social determinants of health are determinants for a reason: they can either create or impair health and well-being based on how much or how little determinants one might have. All determinants of health be it food, housing, transportation, income, education, the environment, etc. are critical. Addressing the social determinants of health typically sits outside of the confines of traditional healthcare structures although its consequences are frequently addressed from within the traditional health structures. It is widely known that many of the manifestations of disease, disability, and mortality are causally linked to the social determinants of health. The artificial boundary with tertiary health care on the one side and the social determinants of health on the other is slowly (and far too slowly in my opinion) being deconstructed. In the United States, we see escalating healthcare costs, increased disease burden, and decreased life expectancy which should be appalling to the sensibilities of any agency/organization or individual whose primary work is to care about health. From a lens of justice in health, health care would be reconciled within a system that embeds the "treatment" of the determinants as a seamless part of its fabric and prioritizes it as part of the mission of that system.

Over 20 years ago, one organization began grappling with unifying the social determinant of health within a health system through a program called *Health Leads* (www.healthleadsusa.org). Health Leads was founded on a vision of standardizing the integration of addressing the social determinants of health within health care. Through partnership across sectors, community-based organizations, and the community of need, Health Leads holistically attends to health needs of the individual within social determinants of health orientation. Importantly, they were able to provide a crucial roadmap capturing the essential and necessary elements that make this approach work. Included in the roadmap are resources and tools related to identification and screening; navigation and resource connection; social health team and workflow; community partnerships, data and evaluation and leadership; and change management (https://healthleadsusa.org/resource-library/roadmap/). Furthermore, they created a compendium of relevant resources and established a network of colleagues and partners who are leading in this space across the United States to promote collective learning, exchange, and progress (https://healthleadsusa.org/network/). Health Leads uses an inclusive approach to addressing the social determinants of health that are most hindering an individual's ability to be healthy and achieve well-being. They leave the door open for other providers and institutions to learn how best to do this within their own communities with an array of tools and resources and networks.

Other organizations choose to tackle social issues and health drivers by mining innovative thought leaders from across the United States to intellectually unearth these persistent patterns of injustice and generate solutions. A leading player in this space is the Aspen Institute (www.aspeninstitute.org). The Aspen Institute is a think tank of innovators, scholars, and creatives who source their ideas for use in solving complex social justice issues, most of which are inequities in relation to the social determinants of health. They charge their constituents to make an impact that improves the human condition locally and globally through a variety of programs, groups, initiatives, and fellowships.

There are innumerable organizations that focus on specific social and structural drivers of health to move the needle along in their community. Food insecurity and economic disparity are fundamental health drivers and determinants which underlay many disease manifestations and stifle opportunity.

Many communities address food insecurity through food pantries which are a necessary emergency intervention and source of survival for families in crisis. Healthy food is foundational to achieving health—the justice making occurs when access to healthy food happens equitably with intention across the spectrum of food access from farm to table.

4.4.1 Community Exemplar: Food Justice Network

Cultivate Charlottesville (cultivatecharlottesville.org) takes an integrated systems approach to build equitable and sustainable food system in their community. According to the network "Cultivate Charlottesville engages youth and community in building an equitable, sustainable food system through garden-based experiential learning, growing and sharing healthy food, amplifying community leaders, and advocating for food justice" (https://cultivatecharlottesville.org/mission/#). This approach posits access to healthy food as an issue of justice based on the belief that food is a human right and access to it has been inequitable. In particular, the network "considers food related health disparities across race and class as non-random outcomes of discriminatory policies" (https://cultivatecharlottesville.org/what-is-food-equity/).

Cultivate Charlottesville created an integrated network of food equity programs and initiatives to coordinate efforts to build healthy and nutritious food accessibility across critical junctures of the overall food system. Their intentional alignment of efforts to align strategies to "amplify impact" is fundamental to justice.

Access to economic opportunity and mobility in the form of wealth creation and wealth generation can be a remedying opportunity to bolster the social determinants of health and their accompanying disparities. Health disparities are subsidized by several factors of which income plays a critical role. The connection between diminished health outcomes and poverty are well established in the literature (Benfer et al., 2019; Brown et al., 2019; Price et al., 2018). This makes economic injustice and the access to opportunity a health issue and the rectification of this chasm a demonstration of health justice. We would be hard pressed to find health science schools and specialties orienting their practitioners in the added value of investing in economic development and social innovation as a health intervention for disparate populations. As radical as this may sound, consideration of economic thriving as a mitigating strategy to buffer poverty by creating wealth and opportunity demands examination. Before unpacking what this engagement by the health sector in this space could look like, I offer the exemplar below to help contextualize this concept.

4.4.2 Community Exemplar: The Russell Innovation Center for Entrepreneurs (RICE)

The Russell Innovation Center for Entrepreneurs (https://russellcenter.org/) was founded to honor and expand the Herman Russell Legacy of successful Black entrepreneurship. As such, it focuses exclusively on Black entrepreneurship as a mechanism to build Black wealth and prosperity in the Black community. They have created an economic ecosystem built on critical supports essential for Black entrepreneurial success using their "big ideas" model (found at https://russellcenter.org/big-ideas/). The IDEAS (Initiate, Develop, Execute, Accelerate and Scale) model guides entrepreneur education, mentorship, access to opportunity, and capital resources using a human-centered approach. Within this model, an economic ecosystem is created that supports Black entrepreneurial pursuits by building a sense of community and intentional networks of access—access to information, access to education, and access to opportunity.

Components of the RICE big IDEAS model (https://russellcenter.org/big-ideas/) refer to the following stages:

- *Inspire stage* is a "safe place to explore curiosities about entrepreneurship and strengthen the entrepreneurial mindset. It is where the entrepreneurial pathway begins and the entrepreneur will establish their big idea, develop a business plan and identify their target customer."
- *Develop stage* is critical to overall business success and "where entrepreneurs will lay the building blocks for the next stages. It is where they will perform a detailed analysis of the problem they are trying to solve, identify and test the market, and assess the level of demand by completing a customer discovery process; developing a working business model and establishing a minimal viable product or service."
- *Execute stage* is the doing and implementation of their business model. It is where discovery of what is possible and feasible comes to life.
- *Accelerate stage* is the "marathon that helps build a stronger business model. This is where entrepreneurs must change the pace, plan for scale and manage risk. It is where the entrepreneur prepares their business to take on high-growth opportunities in various markets."

- Scale stage is achieved by entrepreneurs who "demonstrate a deep knowledge of their customers and markets while achieving strong traction become RICE Pacesetter companies across the Big IDEAS continuum." They become deeply embedded in community building and are "assigned a quarterback coach to help solve problems, access important resources, and keep them connected" (Russell Innovation Center for Entrepreneurs, 2021. Retrieved from: https://russellcenter.org/big-ideas/).

The RICE model offers wrap-around sequential support to target success of Black business owners. It provides anticipatory guidance and structures to help entrepreneurs overcome known pitfalls increasing opportunity for sustained wealth building. Creating sustained wealth building of Black businesses can catalyze generational wealth building potentially staving off poverty by promoting greater access to resources which multiply into positive life options such as better education, healthy foods, improved housing options, and access to capital that can be used to build more capital. The economic equalization spurred by wealth creation among historically economically excluded communities and the subsequent health and wellness benefits is equity and justice.

4.4.3   Community Exemplar: Communities United

Communities United (communitiesunitied.org): takes a community mobilization approach by amplifying the impact of the collective through the development of grassroots leaders whose mission is to achieve "racial justice and transformative change" in focal areas of "advancing affordable housing, health equity, education justice, youth investment, immigrant rights, and advancing public health solutions to community safety" (https://communitiesunited.org/our-mission). This compilation of issues provides a diverse platform to build and focus collective efforts. This exemplar is most poignant because it recognizes that attaining equity and justice involves the intentional engagement of intersecting issues and those closest to the issues. It is a prime demonstration of social innovation and thought leadership that engages various actors to co-create solutions that are sparked by imagination and fueled passion and compassion for more just and equitable health outcomes. Expertise of those with lived experience who are closely connected to experiences within affected communities are valued and given the appropriate respect as the primary generator for solutions. Hence their organizing occurs within the community. They foster and create solutions within and by the communities. Many of their efforts and accomplishments are documented on their website with some extracted below:

- Creating the nation's most comprehensive statewide reform of school discipline policy (SB100), which ended zero-tolerance practices at all publicly funded state schools, placed stronger limits on the use of exclusionary discipline and laid the foundation for the expansion of restorative justice. This sweeping change was led by Voices of Youth in Chicago Education (VOYCE), a core youth-organizing initiative of CU that is led by young people of color.

- Building political will to expand resources for mental health counselors, restorative justice, and other trauma-informed supports for students in schools/districts of highest need to further dismantle the school-to-prison pipeline through the Rethinking Safety campaign, which was adopted as an initiative of the same name by the Illinois legislature in May 2019.
- Effecting groundbreaking policy change at the city level through the Keep Chicago Renting coalition, which increased rights for tenants living in foreclosed properties by requiring foreclosing owners to either renew a tenant's rental agreement or provide $10,600 in relocation assistance.
- Preserving affordable housing (over 400 units are in the pipeline to date) and protecting the rights of renters in foreclosed buildings through successful organizing efforts. This resulted in the City of Chicago creating the Preserving Existing Affordable Rentals (PEAR) program, modeled after ROOTS, and pledging an initial $10 million in funding over 5 years to support.
- Working with other groups to inform Chicago's consent decree on policing to ensure that the needs of people of color with disabilities, including survivors of gun violence, were included.
- Co-convening Healthy Communities in Cook County (HC3) coalition to increase access to health care through the county-level policy change that created a direct-access program for the uninsured, including the undocumented. This was done through an alliance-building approach in which we engaged 40 organizations and over 1000 residents and provided access to health care to over 10,000 uninsured people across Cook County. (Communities United, n.d. Retrieved from https://communitiesunited.org/about-us/what-we-have-done).

Just recently, a new community grassroots foundation was created in partnership with Natrona Collective Health Trust (NCHT) and FSG to engage and listen to community voices to develop a community-informed and community-implemented regional health equity strategy.(https://www.pacesconnection.com/blog/how-a-new-foundation-utilized-community-voice-in-their-strategy-formation-fsg-org).

Fundamental to many of these examples are their orientation within a strengths-based and asset-emphasized approach. Each coalition uses the inherent strengths of the community to lay out the pathway for change in practice and policies to the benefit identified by the community. Health justice is achieved because important steps occur. First, the sharing of power and valuing of community expertise is centered; and second, the focus is on resetting injustice while simultaneously setting up improved infrastructure targeted to attain better and more equitable outcomes.

4.5   Infusing Innovation

Innovation has been a necessary component of many scientific and technological advances in health care and elsewhere. However, it has been less enthusiastically sought after to remedy the social determinants of health until recently with the emergence of social innovation and the expectation associated with reimaging and re-envisioning norms amidst disturbing social unrest and our neo-COVID society. Social innovation is defined as "new ideas that work in meeting social goals" (Mulgan, p. 8). By nature, it is not a new concept. It is one that has had a long-standing historical presence at the heart of many social, economic, and political movements such as civil rights, waves of feminist movements, digital economies, and now the meta-universe.

We have also seen the result of innovation in creating structures, entities, and enterprises ranging from the formation of unions, universal health care, microfinance, and anti-oppression movements. This innovation is channeled toward social advancement and justice making because it is used to fuel priorities that are influenced by context and conditions that exist within it. Social innovation is dynamic in relation to the social environment. Understanding social innovation is to know "that social innovations comprise new ways of doing (practices, technologies, material commitments), organizing (rules, decision-making, modes of governance), framing (meaning, visions, imaginaries, discursive commitments) and knowing (cognitive resources, competence, learning, appraisal)" (Pel et al., 2020, p. 3).

Now we see social innovation gaining traction in the pandemic era, where real-time changes, adaptability, and flexibility were essential to sustaining the most basic of societal functioning. At the height of COVID, the nation simultaneously experienced all-time lows. We were faced with confronting a succession of undeniable truths: truths of a country deeply fractured by its racist history and unreconciled racist structures; truths of the burden of health disparities paid for on the backs of Black, Brown, First Nations, and the poor; truths of the intentional devaluing and killing of Black bodies; truths of inequity in income and access to the most basic of resources of human existence; truths of failures to provide families with a living wage; truths in supply chain and logistical infrastructure insufficiencies; truths of the ramifications of persistent divestment in public health; truths of a system of care on the verge of collapse during COVID-19; and truths of the fragility of our democracy.

Structurally, morally, mentally, and physically the country and the world simultaneously faced existential threats to our existence as we know it. The emergence of innovation was actively sought after as both a reaction and a solution to this tsunami of threats spurring the push for social innovation.

4.5.1 Social Innovation Exemplar: The MacArthur Foundation

The MacArthur Foundation uses research and ingenuity to drive change, articulating their work as "striving to make transformative change in areas of profound concern" (https://www.macfound.org/our-work). The standard used by the institute to do this work is informed by their "Just Imperative" that they described as follows:

Justice is reflected in fairness, equity, impartiality, respect, and humanity, and char-
acterized by the promotion of, and elimination of the past and present barriers to,
equitable access, treatment, consideration, and opportunity.
The Just Imperative requires that we interrogate our decisions and actions to ensure
that they enhance the conditions in which justice can thrive; rejecting and challenging the structures, systems, and practices that reinforce an unjust status quo,
or produce unjust outcomes. (The MacArthur Foundation, 2022b. Retrieved
from https://www.macfound.org/about/how-we-work/just-imperative).

There are similarities in the MacArthur Foundation's The Just Imperative and the
essence of Just Health that primarily align with the expectations of action, self-
reflection, and structural reformation. Health sovereignty would add to this as the
emancipation of the individual's autonomy over their health to achieve the ultimate
fullness of human flourishing.

The MacArthur Foundation channels resources aligned with intelligence and
ingenuity around big bet initiatives—the seemingly impossible behemoth social
challenges and enduring commitments to implement The Just Imperative (https://
www.macfound.org/about/how-we-work/). They mobilize research networks, fel-
lows, fund impact investments, and other philanthropic approaches to address societal issues with urgency. The MacArthur Foundation has prioritized their energy to
tackle the most concerning existential threats of our time such as climate change,
nuclear risk, criminal justice reform, and corruption—the big bets (https://www.
macfound.org/pages/about-our-big-bets).

Justice in health requires taking on our own set of big bets—those areas that create profound obstacles to health sovereignty. This could be a highly subjective offering of what those might be; however, it is felt that in addition to the social determinant
of health, access to health care would rise to the top of that or any other list of barriers to care, health, and flourishing. Unlike the big bets proposed by the MacArthur
Foundation, there are many configurations and models of what access to health care
could look like in the United States. These models could be modified and adopted
to provide a foundational level of universal health care for all Americans.

4.6 Access to Care and Opportunity: Community of Caring

One of the most prolific barriers to health, a known and evidenced accomplice to
health disparities, is the access to health care. Access to care happens when individuals cannot get the health care that they need in its most basic and essential of
forms. Access to opportunity happens when individuals can get equitable access to
those determinants that impact their ability to be healthy and to have longevity.
Access to care and access to opportunity can be democratized by building a community of caring that ensures personal health autonomy and empowered health
determination. Creating a community of care begins with valuing such a sense of
community where compassion to provide care, face historical truths, and ensure

equity in all we do is entrenched and solidified in our practice, actions, systems and structures. Structural reconfiguration that stands up to the ability of the system to be responsive to such a provocative ideal would require principles of universality and a shared equity vision that harmonizes services and increases impact. Universal health care promotes access to care at many system contact points, across many measures that determine health, fostering a care community. Universal access to health is outlined in one of the many targets of the Sustainable Development Goals (https://sdgs.un.org/goals). The Sustainable Development Goals are, in essence, a global social contract for peace and prosperity that were adopted in 2015 by the United Nations around 17 action areas (See Appendix A) to advance equity and ensure better outcomes for the planet, people, and society by 2030 (United Nations Department of Economic and Social Affairs, n.d.). These goals have been adopted by all members of the United Nations and are composed of 17 measures, 169 targets, and 6439 actions (https://sdgs.un.org/goals). The action areas attempt to set an international standard of acceptable social and environmental progress for the world. By adopting these goals, UN member countries are not only endorsing them but committing to their actualization. An important measure among many others within the sustainable development goals is Target 3.8 of these goals. This target aims to "achieve universal health coverage, including financial risk protection, access to quality essential health care services and access to safe, effective, quality and affordable essential medicines and vaccines for all" (WHO, 2022). Entertaining the attainment of this aim unilaterally across the United States presents the rationale and opportunity for a national health policy approach to achieve universal health coverage. The fact that the United States is a signatory to these goals and these goals interface with the United States Healthy People 2030 Goals is significant.

Healthy People 2030 (https://health.gov/healthypeople) is the US Department of Health and Human Services' prioritized goals for health comprising 355 public health objectives and leading health action indicators that focus on the social determinants of health to improve health and well-being. Its overarching aim is to advance health equity (https://health.gov/healthypeople/priority-areas), defined as "the attainment of the highest level of health for all people. Achieving health equity requires valuing everyone equally with focused and ongoing societal efforts to address avoidable inequalities, historical and contemporary injustices, and the elimination of health and health care disparities" (Office of Disease Prevention and Health Promotion, Office of the Assistant Secretary for Health, Office of the Secretary, U.S. Department of Health and Human Services, n.d.) (see Fig. 4.2).

To advance health equity, Healthy People 2030 objectives cover five overarching goals of health conditions, health behaviors, settings and systems, populations, and the social determinants of health. In fact, the social determinants are one of the Healthy People 2030 goals.

As an example to demonstrate justice in health through health policy, the overarching social determinants of health goals and its five objectives, economic stability; education access and quality; healthcare access and quality; neighborhood and built environment; and social and community context from Healthy People 2030 are summatively explored. Each of these social determinants of health objectives have

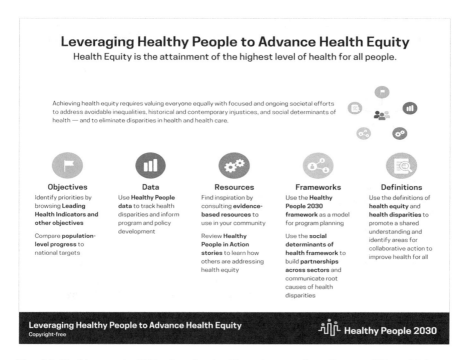

Fig. 4.2 Healthy people 2030 advancing health equity overview. (Source: Office of Disease Prevention and Health Promotion, Office of the Assistant Secretary for Health, Office of the Secretary, U.S. Department of Health and Human Services, n.d. Retrieved from: https://health.gov/healthypeople/priority-areas/health-equity-healthy-people-2030)

a series of very specific indicators used to measure progress on that particular objective. For a more robust dive into each of these five objectives and their series of indicators, please visit the healthypeople.gov website. For now, the objective with part of its rationale and a sample of one of its existing indicators that have been touched upon during our examination of justice in health and are offered to provide educational insight into the intention and opportunity presented by Healthy People 2030.

Objective 1: Economic Stability: *This objective has one goal and nine indicators to help people earn steady incomes that allow them to meet their health needs.*

Rationale: Healthy People 2030 identify that "In the United States, 1 in 10 people live in poverty,1 and many people can't afford things like healthy foods, health care, and housing" (https://health.gov/healthypeople/objectives-and-data/browse-objectives/economic-stability).

Sample Indicator: Reduce the proportion of people living in poverty—SDOH-01.

Objective 2: Education Access and Quality: *This objective has 1 goal and 12 indicators to increase educational opportunities and help children and adolescents do well in school.*

Rationale: Healthy People 2030 identify that "people with higher levels of education are more likely to be healthier and live longer." Children from low-income families, children with disabilities, and children who routinely experience forms of social discrimination—like bullying—are more likely to struggle with math and reading. "They're also less likely to graduate from high school or go to college. This means they're less likely to get safe, high-paying jobs and more likely to have health problems like heart disease, diabetes, and depression" (https://health.gov/healthypeople/objectives-and-data/browse-objectives/education-access-and-quality).

Sample Indicator: Increase interprofessional prevention education in health professions training programs—ECBP-D08.

Objective 3: Healthcare Access and Quality: *This objective has 1 goal and 50 indicators to increase access to comprehensive, high-quality healthcare services.*

Rationale: Healthy People 2030 identify that "about 1 in 10 people in the United States don't have health insurance.1 People without insurance are less likely to have a primary care provider, and they may not be able to afford the health care services and medications they need. Strategies to increase insurance coverage rates are critical for making sure more people get important health care services, like preventive care and treatment for chronic illnesses" (https://health.gov/healthypeople/objectives-and-data/browse-objectives/health-care-access-and-quality).

Sample Indicator: Increase the proportion of adults who get recommended evidence-based preventive health care—AHS-08.

Objective 4: Neighborhood and Built Environment: *This objective has 1 goal and 29 indicators to create neighborhoods and environments that promote health and safety.*

Rationale: Healthy People 2030 identify "the neighborhoods people live in have a major impact on their health and well-being" and that "many people in the United States live in neighborhoods with high rates of violence, unsafe air or water, and other health and safety risks. Racial/ethnic minorities and people with low incomes are more likely to live in places with these risks. In addition, some people are exposed to things at work that can harm their health, like secondhand smoke or loud noises" (https://health.gov/healthypeople/objectives-and-data/browse-objectives/neighborhood-and-built-environment).

Sample Indicator: Reduce the proportion of families that spend more than 30 percent of income on housing—SDOH-04.

Objective 5: Social and Community Context: *This objective has 1 goal and 13 indicators to increase social and community support.*

Rationale: Health People 2030 identify that "people's relationships and interactions with family, friends, co-workers, and community members can have a major impact on their health and well-being." And "many people face challenges and dangers they can't control — like unsafe neighborhoods, discrimination, or trouble affording the things they need. This can have a negative impact on health and safety throughout life. Positive relationships at home, at work, and in the com-

munity can help reduce these negative impacts." (https://health.gov/healthypeo-ple/objectives-and-data/browse-objectives/social-and-community-context).
Sample Indicator: Increase the proportion of adults who talk to friends or family about their health—HC/HIT-04.

Health policy is a tool for building justice in health and to ensure its access. While new policies are needed to fill policy gaps to create health equity, there are many health policies that exist where justice in health can support implementation strategies to enact those policies more effectively and equitably. Review of the indicators provides well-intended action items for organizations and health institutions to focus on. What is absent is understanding how those organizations are encouraged to adopt these goals and indicators as part of their own implementation strategies. A clear impetus beyond the altruistic, i.e., it's the right thing to do to decrease prevalence, could not be found. This leaves the opportunity for the option to either engage with the goals and indicators through programs and initiatives targeting them specifically, or not to engage with Healthy People 2030 at all.

These policy goals demonstrate that there is some sense of a national commitment toward the achievement of health equity and that the issue is known and monitored. What is less clear is the implementation strategy to ensure the achievement of its outcomes and accountability that engagement with its objectives happen. Barriers to care and potential threats to health and the successful achievement of the plan's indicators should be a functional part of any plan. They are potential challenges that have to be identified and attended to in order to facilitate the success of Healthy People 2030.

Prevention services, routine care, examinations, and diagnostic tests are health rights that can be afforded to every human being and are encouraged as part of this much wider global and national agenda. Chapter 1 examined the conversation about health as a right, and access to care is where this right is evident or not. Having insurance does not mean that an individual has access to care. The type of insurance, the coverage limits, and co-payments can render the insured, either under-insured or reluctant, to use the insurance given the high levels of out-of-pocket costs that will be incurred. The location of healthcare services determines access. An individual may live in rural and remote areas where healthcare services are not nearby and travel is an obstacle to being able to see a primary care provider, if there are any in the area. Those in urban spaces may be nearer to hospitals however may use those services as a safety net for primary healthcare services and have transportation challenges (not having money for parking or having to take public transportation) that inhibit their ability to get to the hospital. Furthermore, disparate populations in most need of health care could be lower wage workers who cannot afford taking time off work to go to the hospital or see their healthcare provider. Communities with historical distrust of medical providers outright refuse to seek care at all, given the history of exploitation by the medical community or are subjected to substandard care evidenced along lines of race and marginalized identities.

What is most obnoxiously disturbing about this issue is that it is an issue happening in one of the wealthiest nations in the world. How have we gotten to a place where access to health care is still such a significant problem that literally costs people their lives yet is allowed to persist? Chapter 5 will dive deeper into systems of care and what a reimagined system could look like. It pushes exploration about what our system could look like and asks how do we make it happen? Health happens in many spaces and any configured system should account for the variability of health needs within the various contexts of health care. All these considerations lead us back to the initial question on what health is and why a shared understanding of health is absolutely critical to the ways in which we operationalize and allocate health care in the United States. The justice making of health occurs when we lead with this shared understanding as a core value reflected in our actions that include our provider education and training, ease and scope of access to services (preventative and tertiary), and lives of those who need it most. Living our Justice in Health imperative becomes a natural and ecological occurrence that is prioritized unilaterally in all decisions related to the human condition.

4.7   Conclusion: Revisiting the Story of Donell and Tonya

In the case of both Tonya and Donell, the following questions were posed:

1. Although Tonya is being treated for diabetes, what other health issues need attending to that influence her chronic condition? Where is the disconnect here?
2. Although Donell is being treated for hypertension, what other health issues need attending to that influence his chronic condition? Where is the disconnect here?

In both cases, the client is being treated for the presenting condition with a hyperfocus on the disease and not the conditions that sustain and optimize health. While it is not unusual for healthcare providers to focus on the "treatment," it cannot continue to be the sole driver to provide care, irrespective of setting. Physical assessments and diagnosis of disease and other conditions are required, and it is not being suggested that they discontinue. It is being suggested that these sorts of assessments should not be idolized as the exclusive determining factor of health. A health justice perspective would expect that any patient who presents at any point of entry into a health system be assessed comprehensively for all health-related issues that are presented and not presented. Even further, the lion share of healthcare system action cannot be reactive and passively assume a wait and see posture, where the patient is seen when the patient shows up for care.

The Tonya's and Donell's of such a scenario may not be able to show up until it's too late and disease has manifested to the point that costly medical intervention is now required. Worse, they may not be able to show up at all. What could have been prevented with early intervention was not simply because the healthcare system was complicit in implementing a prevention mandate that served to quell the progression of disease. An effective prevention mandate uses a multi-pronged approach of health promotion, outreach, education, screening, and connecting families with resources. The disconnect in Tonya and Donell started with failing to integrate their unique context into the plan of care and treat the conditions and the disease simultaneously.

The justice in health orientation is critical in these situations because it exacts the point that health is not the absence of disease, but instead a spectrum of interrelated conditions that must be assuaged to achieve human flourishing the truest form of well-being. This is not only the intention of the United Nations Sustainable Development Goals but also appears to be the case for the United States Healthy People 2030. What is required to make the targets national and contribute to the successful achievement of targets globally is what must be overcome next. Human flourishing cannot produce well-being without structural rectification of the system of health, the fundamental beliefs about health, and the democratization of health.

Appendices

Appendix A: Sustainable Development Goals (SDGs) (United Nations Department of Economic and Social Affairs, n.d.)

1. **End poverty in all its forms everywhere:** This goal's targets attend to creating opportunity and economic and policy infrastructure to achieve self-sufficiency and decrease incidence of poverty.
2. **Zero Hunger: End hunger, achieve food security and improved nutrition and promote sustainable agriculture**: This indicator targets decreasing hunger and malnutrition with a focus on upstanding and investing in equity and sustainable food systems and agricultural practices.
3. **Good Health and Well Being: Ensure healthy lives and promote well-being for all at all ages.** This goal is aimed at maternal child health, communicable and noncommunicable disease, substance use, injury prevention and health system access, and workforce.
4. **Quality Education:** Ensure inclusive and equitable quality education and promote lifelong learning opportunities for all.
5. **Gender Equality:** Achieve gender equality and empower all women and girls.
6. **Clean Water and Sanitation:** Ensure availability and sustainable management of water and sanitation for all.
7. **Affordable and Clean Energy:** Ensure access to affordable, reliable, sustainable, and modern energy for all.
8. **Decent Work and Economic Growth:** Promote sustained, inclusive, and sustainable economic growth, full and productive employment, and decent work for all.
9. **Industry Innovation and Infrastructure:** Build resilient infrastructure, promote inclusive and sustainable industrialization, and foster innovation.
10. **Reduce inequality:** Reduce inequality within and among countries.
11. **Sustainable Communities and Cities:** Make cities and human settlements inclusive, safe, resilient, and sustainable.
12. **Responsible production and consumption:** Ensure sustainable consumption and production patterns.
13. **Climate Action:** Take urgent action to combat climate change and its impacts.

14. **Life Below Water:** Conserve and sustainably use the oceans, seas, and marine resources for sustainable development.
15. **Life on Land:** Protect, restore, and promote sustainable use of terrestrial ecosystems, sustainably manage forests, combat desertification, and halt and reverse land degradation and halt biodiversity loss.
16. **Peace Justice and Strong Institutions:** Promote peaceful and inclusive societies for sustainable development, provide access to justice for all, and build effective, accountable, and inclusive institutions at all levels.
17. **Partnerships for the Goals:** Strengthen the means of implementation and revitalize the Global Partnership for Sustainable Development.

Appendix B: Selected SDG Progress Updates: Exemplars in Evidence of the Need for Justice in Health

"In 2020, for the first time in two decades, the world's share of workers living with their families below the international poverty line increased from 6.7% in 2019 to 7.2%, pushing an additional 8 million workers into poverty. Although the working poverty rate decreased slightly in 2021 to 6.9%, it was still higher than the pre-pandemic rate" (United Nations Department of Economic and Social Affairs. SDG 1. https://sdgs.un.org/goals/goal1).

"By 2020, only 47% of the global population were effectively covered by at least one social protection cash benefit, leaving 4.1 billion people unprotected. In response to the COVID-19 crisis, more than 1700 social protection measures (mostly short-term) were announced by 209 countries and territories" (United Nations Department of Economic and Social Affairs. SDG 1. https://sdgs.un.org/goals/goal1).

"In 2020, between 720 and 811 million people in the world were suffering from hunger – as many as 161 million more than in 2019." Thirty percent (2.4 billion people) – were moderately or severely food insecure, lacking regular access to adequate food… "an increase of almost 320 million people in just one year" (United Nations Department of Economic and Social Affairs. SDG 2. https://sdgs.un.org/goals/goal2).

References

Banzhaf, S., Ma, L., & Timmins, C. (2019). Environmental justice: The economics of race, place, and pollution. *Journal of Economic Perspectives, 33*(1), 185–208.
Benfer, E. A., Mohapatra, S., Wiley, L. F., & Yearby, R. (2019). Health justice strategies to combat the pandemic: Eliminating discrimination, poverty, and health disparities during and after COVID-19. *Yale Journal of Health Policy, Law, and Ethics, 19*, 122.
Black Lives Matter. (2022). Retrieved May 19, 2022 from: https://blacklivesmatter.com/

Brown, A. F., Ma, G. X., Miranda, J., Eng, E., Castille, D., Brockie, T., Jones, P., Airhihenbuwa, C., Farhat, T., & Trinh-Shevrin, C. (2019). Structural interventions to reduce and eliminate health disparities. *American Journal of Public Health, 109*(S1), S72–S78.

Burnett, C., Ford-Gilboe, M., Berman, H., Ward-Griffin, C., & Wathen, N. (2015). A critical analysis of provincial policies impacting shelter service delivery to women exposed to violence. *Politics, Policy and Nursing Journal, 16*(1–2), 5–16. https://doi.org/10.1177/1527154415583123

Burnett, C., Ford-Gilboe, M., Berman, H., Wathen, N., & Ward-Griffin, C. (2016). Day to day reality of shelter service delivery to abused women in the context of system and policy demands. *Journal of Social Service Research.* https://doi.org/10.1177/1527154415583123

Burnett, C., Swanberg, M., Hudson, A., & Schminkey, D. (2018, Winter). Structural justice: A critical feminist framework exploring the intersection between justice, equity and structural reconciliation. *Journal of Health Disparities Research and Practice, 11*(4), 52–68.

Centers for Disease Control and Prevention. (2019). *ACES vital signs report.* Retrieved from: https://www.cdc.gov/vitalsigns/aces/index.html#:~:text=%20Adverse%20Childhood%20 Experiences%20impact%20lifelong%20health%20and,risk%20for%20health%20 problems%20across%20the...%20More%20

Centers for Disease Control and Prevention. (2021a). *Preventing intimate partner violence fact sheet.* Retrieved July 5, 2022 from: https://www.cdc.gov/violenceprevention/pdf/ipv/IPV-factsheet_2021.pdf

Centers for Disease Control and Prevention. (2021b). CDC Fast Facts Preventing Intimate Partner Violence (2022). Retrieved May 18, 2022 from: https://www.cdc.gov/violenceprevention/inti-matepartnerviolence/fastfact.html

Centers for Disease Control and Prevention. (2021c). *Impact of Racism on our Nation's health,* Retrieved May 17, 2022 from: https://www.cdc.gov/healthequity/racism-disparities/impact-of-racism.html

Centers for Disease Control and Prevention. (2021d). *Racism and health.* Retrieved May 17, 2022 from: https://www.cdc.gov/healthequity/racism-disparities/index.html

Centers for Disease Control and Prevention. (2021e). *CDC vital signs Adverse Childhood Experiences (ACEs) Preventing early trauma to improve adult health (Nov 2019).* https://www.cdc.gov/vitalsigns/aces/pdf/vs-1105-aces-H.pdf

Centers for Disease Control and Prevention. (2022). *National center for injury prevention and control division of violence prevention.* Retrieved July 5, 2022 from: https://www.cdc.gov/violenceprevention/communityviolence/prevention.html

Communities United Retrieved December 17, 2021 from (communitiesunitied.org).

Communities United. (n.d.). *About us.* Retrieved January 8, 2022 from https://communitiesunited.org/about-us/what-we-have-done

Cultivate Charlottesville. (2021a). Retrieved December 12, 2021 from: https://cultivatecharlot-tesville.org/mission/

Cultivate Charlottesville. (2021b). Retrieved December 21, 2021 from: https://cultivatecharlot-teville.org/what-is-food-equity/

Cure Violence. (2021). Retrieved October 2, 2021 from: cvg.org

Do, D. P., Locklar, L. R., & Florsheim, P. (2019). Triple jeopardy: The joint impact of racial segregation and neighborhood poverty on the mental health of black Americans. *Social Psychiatry and Psychiatric Epidemiology, 54*(5), 533–541.

Equal Justice Initiative. (2021). Retrieved October 2, 2021 from: https://eji.org/about/

Ghandnoosh, N. (2015). Black lives matter: Eliminating racial inequity. In *The criminal justice system. The sentencing project research and advocacy reform* (pp. 1–36). Retrieved July 5, 2022 from: https://www.sentencingproject.org/publications/black-lives-matter-eliminating-racial-inequity-in-the-criminal-justice-system/#II.%20A%20Cascade%20of%20Racial%20 Disparities%20Throughout%20the%20Criminal%20Justice%20System

Government. United States. (2022). *S. 3623: Violence against Women Act Reauthorization Act of 2022.* Retrieved May 18, 2022 from: https://www.govtrack.us/congress/bills/117/s3623

Harrell, S. P. (2000). A multidimensional conceptualization of racism-related stress: Implications for the well-being of people of color. *American Journal of Orthopsychiatry, 70*(1), 42–57.

Health Leads. (2021a). Retrieved November 4, 2021 from: www.healthleadsusa.org

Health Leads. (2021b). Retrieved November 4, 2021 from: https://healthleadsusa.org/resource-library/roadmap/

Hicken, M. T., Kravitz-Wirtz, N., Durkee, M., & Jackson, J. S. (2018). Racial inequalities in health: Framing future research. *Social Science & Medicine, 1982*(199), 11–18. https://doi.org/10.1016/j.socscimed.2017.12.027

Kegler, S. R., Simon, T. R., Zwald, M. L., et al. (2022). Vital signs: Changes in firearm homicide and suicide rates — United States, 2019–2020. *MMWR. Morbidity and Mortality Weekly Report, 71*, 656–663. https://doi.org/10.15585/mmwr.mm7119e1externalicon

Mulgan, R (2007). *Social innovation: What it is, why it matters and how it can be accelerated.* Retrieved January 14, 2022 from: https://youngfoundation.org/wp-content/uploads/2012/10/Social-Innovation-what-it-is-why-it-matters-how-it-can-be-accelerated-March-2007.pdf

National Coalition Against Domestic Violence National domestic violence hotline (2022). Retrieved May 18, 2022 from: https://www.thehotline.org/

National Coalition Against Domestic Violence Statistics. (2022a). Retrieved May 18, 2022 from: https://ncadv.org/statistics

National Coalition Against Domestic Violence Statistics. (2022b). Retrieved May 18, 2022 from: https://ncadv.org/

National Network to End Domestic Violence. (2022). Retrieved May 18, 2022 from: https://nnedv.org/

Office of Disease Prevention and Health Promotion, Office of the Assistant Secretary for Health, Office of the Secretary, U.S. Department of Health and Human Services. (n.d.). *Health equity in healthy people 2030*. Healthy People 2030. Retrieved July 9, 2022 from: https://health.gov/healthypeople/priority-areas/health-equity-healthy-people-2030).

Paces Connection. (2022). Retrieved May 18, 2022 from: https://www.pacesconnection.com/blog/how-a-new-foundation-utilized-community-voice-in-their-strategy-formation-fsg-org

Pel, B., Haxeltine, A., Avelino, F., Dumitru, A., Kemp, R., Bauler, T., Kunze, I., Dorland, J., Wittmayer, J., & Jorgensen, M. (2020). Toward a theory of transformative social innovation: A relational framework and 12 propositions. *Research Policy, 49*(8), 1–13. https://doi.org/10.1016/j.respol.2020.104080

Pinchevsky, G. M., & Wright, E. M. (2012). The impact of neighborhoods on intimate partner violence and victimization. *Trauma, Violence, & Abuse, 13*(2), 112–132.

Price, J. H., Khubchandani, J., & Webb, F. J. (2018). Poverty and health disparities: What can public health professionals do? *Health Promotion Practice, 19*(2), 170–174.

Russell Innovation Center for Entrepreneurs. (2021). *Big ideas*. Retrieved October 6 from: https://russellcenter.org/big-ideas/

Singh, S., Archarya, A., Challagundla, K., & Byrareddy, S. (2020, July 21). Impact of social determinants of health on the emerging COVID-19 Pandemic in the United States. *Public Health*. https://doi.org/10.3389/fpubh.2020.00406

The MacArthur Foundation. (2022a). Retrieved January 17, 2022 from: https://www.macfound.org/our-work

The MacArthur Foundation. (2022b). *The just imperative*. Retrieved January 17, 2022 from: https://www.macfound.org/about/how-we-work/just-imperative

The United States Government. Department of Health and Human Services. (2022). *Healthy people 2030*. Retrieved July 9, 2022 from: https://health.gov/healthypeople

The Young Foundation. (2022). Retrieved from: https://youngfoundation.org/wp-content/uploads/2012/10/Social-Innovation-what-it-is-why-it-matters-how-it-can-be-accelerated-March-2007.pdf

United Nations Department of Economic and Social Affairs. (n.d.). *The sustainable development goals*. Retrieved August 30, 2022 from: https://sdgs.un.org/goals

Violence Interrupters. (2022). Retrieved May 18, 2022 from: https://www.violenceinterrupters.org/

World Health Organization. (2022). Retrieved July 5, 2022 from: https://www.who.int/data/gho/data/themes/topics/indicator-groups/indicator-group-details/GHO/sdg-target-3.8-achieve-universal-health-coverage-(uhc)-including-financial-risk-protection

Chapter 5
Culture of Healing

This chapter starts to explore how to create a healthcare system without walls. This chapter reframes the current beliefs of what a healthcare system is, toward what it could be within the concept of building a system of care without walls. A healthcare system without walls is discussed by identifying structural obstacles and gaps within the current structure including their impacts and introducing new ways to overcome and dismantle these challenges.

A core pillar in this discussion is critical conversations about what it means to be a healthcare provider and how we can better prepare healthcare providers to meet the demands of a new reimagined system. To this end, the chapter also introduces trauma-informed approaches, one of the key professional shifts required in the routine preparation of healthcare providers. As an overarching mechanism for facilitating healing, this chapter covers understanding trauma, its consequences, and its impacts at an individual and community level. It examines what a culture of healing looks like through a trauma-informed orientation and explores the healing of individuals and communities who have experienced trauma. The core elements of a trauma-informed approach and their application across this spectrum include recommendations and useful approaches to implementing a culture of healing are provided.

5.1 Reimagination

Reimagining what US health care can be requires, at its core, philosophical shifts in what we believe health to be, why we believe that is what health is, and how can health be attainable for all. Fundamental to unpacking our beliefs is also seeking to understand the ideology shaping the current healthcare system and how it appears through our policy, politics, and values. These are then reflected by healthcare resource and service allocation, healthcare stakeholders and actors' practices and engagement, and the outcomes of all of these combined.

Health care is a political, and increasingly deeply partisan issue that is configured in a revenue exchange system of stakeholders that drives a significant portion of costs through complex reimbursements that are dominated by a fee-for-service payer model. The system reflects a structure that embeds financial drivers with intricate reimbursement formulas for fee exchanges with entities heavily invested in the industry of health care such as pharmaceutical companies and insurance companies and hospitals. This largely impacts hospital billing, service provider and pharmaceutical costs, and consumer costs making it a significant driver of and influencer in the configuration of our system of care. With this influence, the United States spends more of its GDP than any OECD nation on health care yet has the worst health outcomes of all of those nations. While the United States spent about 18% of its GDP on health care (Papanicolas, Woskie, and Jha, 2018); other countries spent much less of their GDP on health care, ranging from 9% in Australia to 12% in Switzerland, despite having more than 99% of their populations covered (Florimon, 2019; Rosso, 2021). Life expectancy in the United States continues to decline, obesity is at an all-time high, and maternal and infant mortality is higher (Florimon, 2019).

The cost of pharmaceutical medication continues to be expensive (Peter G Foundation, 2019) and the average physician earning in the United States is high (Weatherby Healthcare, 2021). The United States is unique among developed countries in that it does not safeguard its citizens against unfair prescription medicine pricing and overcharging. Japan, Taiwan, the United Kingdom, Germany, and Switzerland have all negotiated cheaper rates for brand-name pharmaceuticals on behalf of their citizens with pharmaceutical companies (Palfreman, 2008). Citizens in these countries pay significantly less for prescription pharmaceuticals because of the negotiated prices, which greatly reduces the total medical expenditure in these countries. A patient prescription price review was done in Japan and Taiwan to enforce restrictions that regulate the maximum cost at which manufacturers can sell brand-name drugs and to also negotiate a cap at which companies can sell brand and generic drugs. This negotiation between the government and the drug companies has devised a pricing system for brand-name pharmaceuticals that is on average 35–40% cheaper than in the United States (Palfreman, 2008; De Lew & Greenberg, 1992).

In 2018, pharmaceutical firms and their trade partners spent around $220 billion lobbying in the United States (Scutti, 2019). Even though countries understand the serious challenges created by high prescription drug prices, little has been accomplished in the United States in terms of regulatory or legislative reform of the pharmaceutical and healthcare industry. Prescription drug costs are out of control, with rising cost of prescription pharmaceuticals posing additional problems for patients. Due to high out-of-pocket prices, around 25% of Americans find it difficult to afford prescription medications. High drug prices, according to drug corporations, are critical for supporting innovation (Blumenthal et al., 2021). However, the power to demand exorbitant costs for each new drug may stifle innovation.

During President Joe Biden's 2022 State of the Union speech, he emphasized the problems with high cost of prescription drugs in America, stating that "we pay more for the same drug, produced by the same company in America, than any other country in the world" (State of the Union – Biden, 2022). President Biden further highlighted how expensive the cost of insulin is and how many Americans depend on insulin to live daily because of diabetes by sharing the story of Joshua Davis and his dad who have diabetes. "Insulin costs $10 dollars a vial to make, pharmaceutical companies charge Joshua and his dad up to thirty times that amount" (State of the Union - Biden, 2022). Imagine being Joshua's parents and carrying the ongoing stress of finding ways to pay for necessary life-saving medications. This is what millions of Americans deal with every day. They are in desperate need of these costly medications but have to weigh the options of purchasing their medication with other needs like rent, clothing, food, utilities, and gas. Many Americans end up having to "choose" to neglect or compromise their health because they must prioritize other bills and must first meet their basic needs, which eventually forces them back to the same system to seek urgent care and, worse, end up paying the ultimate price with their lives.

Given that the US healthcare system is set up within a limited health insurance structure, private health insurance continues to be a major obstacle in the healthcare system. There are currently about 50 million people and households, which also include seven million undocumented immigrants who do not have health insurance (KFF analysis, 2021). When a major health event happens, it can be expensive for the uninsured and under-insured. Even before the event, not accessing preventative services also creates and exacerbates health issues. Costs of health care and insurance premiums are rising much faster than inflation (Archer, 2019).

Countries like Japan and Taiwan have all their citizens covered comprehensively and exclusively by either national medical insurance for the self-employed or social insurance for employees. Co-payments are capped depending on one's income and if a job is lost, people do not lose their health insurance, because they are automatically switched to a community insurance plan (Nomura & Nakayama, 2005; Wu et al., 2010). The Taiwanese government before 1995 mirrored their insurance system like the United States. There was a patchwork of different healthcare coverages covering some of the population causing loopholes, then they introduced the National Health Insurance (NHI) system in 1995, (Wu et al., 2010, Palfreman, 2008) to integrate all the different healthcare coverages into a single national insurance system. Their primary objectives were to improve the effectiveness and efficiency of the Taiwanese healthcare coverage system and to make health care more equitable for all citizens, not just rich or more privileged citizens (Wu et al., 2010). Every Taiwanese citizen has a National Health Insurance card which is used to identify a person's medical history and bill the national insurer, funded on tax revenue from employees, employers, and the local and national government. As of 2020, Taiwan spends about 6.2% of its gross domestic product on health care, while the United States spends about 19.7% (Wu et al., 2010; Yang, 2022). Taiwan is just one country example that offers another perspective and evidence that there are viable alternatives to the current approach being used in the United States.

In Canada, health care is provided in all 10 provinces and 13 territories affirmed through the Canadian Health Act of the Federal Government which "establishes criteria and conditions for health insurance plans that must be met by provinces and territories in order for them to receive full federal cash transfers in support of health" (Government of Canada, 2019). These provinces and territories are "required to provide reasonable access to medically necessary hospital and doctors' services" (Government of Canada, 2019) and are given cash and tax transfers for health through the Canada Health Transfer. The costs of this publicly funded health are generated through federal, provincial, and territorial tax revenue, "such as personal and corporate taxes, sales taxes, payroll levies etc…" (Government of Canada, 2019) in addition to federal government equalization payments. The Canada Health Act of 1984 consolidated the principles of previous federal hospital and medical insurance acts into five criteria for health coverage: portability, accessibility, universality, comprehensiveness, and public administration (Government of Canada, 2019). Martin et al. (2018) discuss the criteria and their meanings as:

–   Public administration: plans must be administered and operated on a non-profit basis by a public authority.
–   Comprehensiveness: plans must cover all insured health services provided by hospitals, physicians, or dentists (for surgical dental procedures that require a hospital setting).
–   Universality: all insured residents must be entitled to the insured health services on uniform terms and conditions.
–   Portability: insured residents moving from one province or territory to another, or temporarily absent from their home province or territory or Canada, must continue to be covered for insured health services (within certain conditions).
–   Accessibility: not to impede or preclude, either directly or indirectly, whether by user charges or otherwise, reasonable access to insured health services (Martin et al., 2018, p. 1721). They contend that to Canadians, "the notion that access to health care should be based on need, not ability to pay, is a defining national value" (Martin et al., 2018, p. 1718).

COVID-19 spotlighted the extreme fragility of the US healthcare system and its inability to sufficiently perform to capacity. Dangerously, our healthcare system teetered on collapse. While it is understood that COVID is a unique one in a lifetime phenomenon that tested even the best of systems, what makes this so completely unacceptable is that there is no other healthcare system in the world had the head start in terms of healthcare technology, surveillance, state-of-the-art facilities resources, and expertise all in one. We were the best equipped and least able to respond at the level that should be expected from the costliest healthcare system in the world. This failure was fueled by the historical divestment in public health and exorbitant unmet needs in the most vulnerable of populations. While it is understood that each country has its own unique context, there are adoptable policies and lessons to be learned from other countries who have managed to successfully implement a universal strategy. The United States could benefit from humbly examining and using other global exemplars as a starting point for customizing a system solution that fits within our own country context.

5.2   Re-centering Our Care

The mere privilege of providing care to another human being comes with a certain level of responsibility to the consumer of that care. Patient-centered care is the traditional nomenclature used to convey this sentiment. It is central to most provider statements at healthcare service centers and hospitals and deeply rooted in a medical orientation. Patient-centered care is espoused as a practice standard across many healthcare professions; however, applying this standard from a health justice perspective raises more questions and layers of exploration to understand what patient-centered care really means, for whom, and how it occurs?

To provide patient-centered care, there has to be a patient; one that is presumed to enter the system of care in some way. From there the patient receives care that is focused on their presented need and then the level of their satisfaction with that care encounter is determined. According to the American Medical Association, patient-centered care is "the practice of assessing patient-centered care through the lens of care coordination and patient satisfaction (AMA, 2022)." Others have also broadened this notion to include aspects related to patient satisfaction (such as relationship, empathy) and consider coordination of services a key component of patient-centered care. Eklund et al. (2019) conducted a systematic review of patient- and person-centered care examined across 21 studies and found overlap in their themes and differences in their meaning. This study revealed that both patient- and person-centered care entail: (1) empathy, (2), respect (3), engagement, (4), relationship, (5) communication, (6) shared decision-making, (7) holistic focus, (8), individualized focus, and (9) coordinated care (Eklund et al., p. 3). However, they offer differing goals being the goal of person-centered care is a meaningful life, while the goal of patient-centered care is a functional life (Eklund et al., p. 3).

Moving our language and practice from patient-centered to person-centered care connotes a more inclusive view of the whole individual and their unique human experiences. It takes an intersectional view of the person and embraces the multiplicity of their experiences and their identities (Crenshawe, 1991). Person-centered care "refers to a type of care where the care provider focuses on the needs and resources of the patient and can be defined as co-creation of care between the patients, their family, informal care takers, and health professionals" (Pirhonen et al., 2017, p. 169). Furthermore, this type of care has been shown to increase care quality while decreasing the costs of care (Hansson et al., 2016; Pirhonen et al., 2017).

Most healthcare systems are understood first from the purview of the dominant health system service structure and then the consumer (patient) as a guest of the system. Sandwiched somewhere in the middle are the associated mechanisms of care delivery that include technology, providers, decentralized administration, and access to alternate levels of care. The patient who is the consumer of services, infuse this preconfigured structure based on their health status and its fit with the structure (acuity to chronicity); the patient's ability to access care (insurance, transportation, and location); and care costs which are all shaped by their context including their social determinants of health. So, while they are the largest system actors, they have the least amount of influence, power, and control yet absorb the greatest impacts (positive and negative) of the actions of the upper two levels.

To rebuild our healthcare system, the concept must be inverted with the consumers prioritized across a health care continuum supported by an upstream holistic health approach as much as possible. To help advance and expand our current approach to health care, the new health model pyramid is proposed (Fig. 5.1). This new model of health is intentionally inverted to visually depict how to conceptually reimagine the focus of our health system. It is an attempt to simplify a very interrelated yet disconnected system of care that we currently experience. While there are scholars who have written books on the intricacies of the US healthcare system, this chapter is not an attempt to revisit and explain the obvious—that being the system is in need of radical change. To the contrary, we are embarking on reimagining to attempt the daunting but not impossible task of rebuilding the US system of health care founded on health justice.

Health consumers are everyone and considered to be anyone who is or is not actively engaging in what is traditionally viewed as the health system (clinics, hospital, primary care). Health consumers are every individual for whom health happens, everywhere they are and everywhere they go. Reframing everyone as a health consumer allows for health to be thought of outside of and as owned by an institutional structure. It dials back the belief that people have to go somewhere to receive health from some who provide it to them which implies that health is brokered like a commodity. The idea of everyone as health consumers also steers our belief away from one where people who do not have disease and episodes of sickness are categorized as "healthy." Categorizing healthy versus unhealthy in this manner establishes an artificial and false construct of health by relegating it along a definitive line which you are on either one side of or the other. It does not permit the fluidity of health from moment to moment. Nor does it permit health to breathe at a rhythm that allows for autonomy and the consideration of one's environment, culture, and context.

Fig. 5.1 The new health model

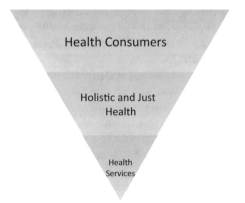

Holistic and just health are integrated approaches that are human-centered, accessible, and equitable inside and outside of structures. This means that everyone must have access to care, universally, and that access should encompass fundamental care services (prevention, screening, required emergency, and routine services) and critical pharmaceuticals to support human health and flourishing. While not comprehensive, this is a place to start, and from there further refinements, inclusion, and modifications can be made.

There are so many ways integrated just and holistic health might look, but if the common understanding is that these are the priority values, then implementation can be flexible and tailored to community and context, acknowledging both are constantly changing. A static system that approaches everyone equally is not proposed. Nor is one that reacts to issues once they are obvious or presented. Instead, a holistic and just system is one that anticipates and removes obstacles to care with more global intent on equitable human flourishing. It is one where the goal is to keep people out of the system versus attending to them within the system. Quality of care is recognized and rewarded based on how well the system facilitates health equity and prevents diseases instead of managing and intervening in the disease amidst health disparity. Human-centered values are embedded and entail the intersectional acceptance of the whole person combined with trauma-informed approach principles toward healthful healing and promotion of thriving across the continuum of life.

At the bottom of the inverted pyramid is the diminished focus on traditional systems as the sole solution and the defining space for health. Health happens in communities, in homes, in families, and within the individual. Its brokering should not be confined to one specific health space, and when this does occur, it should only be at the point of having exhausted all other health avenues and true absolute need in crisis. Tertiary care cannot be a safety net solution and first stop destination for all things health. Hence its size and focus are minimized to reiterate a marked shift in resources, focus, and energy.

5.3   Health as a System Without Walls

What is our system of health care really about? The obvious response is that it is about providing health care, yet what justice in health has shown us is that many layers of unpacking about health need to occur. To truly align our mission with our intention, the exploration around health must start with consensus building around what health is and then executing our resources and energies in that direction. We must start this important process by clearly identifying what the priority goal of a healthcare system should be. A simple interpretation would be to keep people healthy by promoting health and wellness through treatment and prevention. The promotion of health and wellness from prevention to intervention requires the involvement of many key stakeholders at many systems entry points. Several bottlenecks and barriers to access such as distrust, insurance, health literacy (Lazar &

Davenport, 2018), and race/gender/identity (Butkus et al., 2020) exist that we need to overcome.

Recently the American College of Physicians (Butkus et al., 2020) published a position paper proposing "strategies to address social determinants of health and reduce barriers to health to achieve a vision for a better health care system" to achieve a workable and helpful health system. In their vision statement, the American College of Physicians identify the need for a health system that attends to the social determinants of health; adopts a cost structure that redirects dollars to public health, research, and interventions related to the social determinants of health; infuses equity into primary care and other pay structures; and one where systems are incentivized toward improved outcomes, lower costs, and decreasing inequities (Butkus et al., 2020). If achieved, any expectation for success should include at minimum a return on its investment indicative of a system whose investment (resources) do not outperform its benefits (improved health). Oversight and accountability of system actors are key to monitoring and ensuring acceptable performance. Stockbrokers monitor our investments in the market, so *health brokers* should be assigned to monitor the health of the nation, consistently and with full authority to propose modifications that improve performance. Healthcare providers are the life source of our healthcare system; therefore, they need to prepare pre- and post-licensure to service in alignment with the values of a new system. And finally, the values of a new system absolutely must prioritize public health and the determinants of health as part of, and not separate from, health. Doing so would center a holistic view of the patient allowing for a far more coordinated and comprehensive care model that offers basic health rights for all.

We need to create a healthcare system without walls real or perceived. Creating a system without walls starts with valuing the right to health care for all beyond a disease orientation. Health must be understood, enacted holistically, and be accessible and attainable in multiple spaces. There is no room for a reconfigured system based on antiquated beliefs of health as the absence of disease and one that continues to produce increasing health disparities adding further burdens to the entire system. An extremely hard reset of values must occur that involves all players in the current system of care, including its stakeholders and most importantly, its consumers.

Government is the one entity that holds enough position control and regulatory oversight to centrally coordinate and lead the realignment of health values. Advocacy and not-forprofits organizations can also achieve this through coalition-building efforts. Healthcare consumers can exert pressure on the government to orchestrate a new approach to health care. However, to make a seismic shift in the resetting of our healthcare values, narratives around what we believe health to be must change. Intentional dialogues about health can happen just about anywhere, but there must be coordinated agreement, consensus and partnership building, an implementation strategy, and with designated leadership able to lead inspiring action toward system change.

5.4   The Rationale for Justice in Health

COVID-19 has opened the opportunity for a national health dialogue because of the issues and challenges that arose and resurfaced during the pandemic. The ramifications of COVID-19 are still being felt and have played out in healthcare system exhaustion, struggle to recover to pre-COVID service levels, and a healthcare shortage that still impedes our efforts to deliver the most basic levels of care. This is the perfect jumping off point for exploring and implementing deep system reform. It is the ideal moment for the bringing together of thought leaders and thought partners to engage in a national health dialogue with the intention of informing the development of a national strategy to recalibrate and reset our health system.

Using a justice in health lens to stand up a national health dialogue and strategy endorses the shared belief of a common value in health as a right, and one that is situated in a holistic human-centered orientation and advocates for equitable human flourishing of all. These shared values can be the minimum charge and provide an unwavering focus of any design thinking process to re-envisioning our current system. Getting to shared values and beliefs about the right to health to achieve human flourishing must first involve the fundamental philosophical agreement around what health is. Chapter 1 examined the historical narratives around health and provided an evolutionary pathway to enhancing our definition of health. Clarity around the definition of health brings clarity to our decisions around health care. Earlier understanding of health focused on disease which produced a system that is disproportionately and frankly unsustainably orientated around disease and sickness. Moving to clarity in our definition and our shared health values will influence what providing care with a renewed conceptualization of health looks like. Building consensus around health and its provision will warrant the letting go of old health beliefs and making room for new ones. It is the acceptance that these new beliefs will look different and require new approaches that will need to be brought to bear. Territorialism and professional tribalism have no place in a system that is truly focused on a common goal and shared outcome. Likewise, industry interests cannot be put before human interests.

The politics of health care have politicized health and set it up as an ever-present campaign battleground issue generating opposing visions and views of health. Fundamentally both ends of the political spectrum agree that people should have health care, the difference is in how that should occur. If the belief is that the most basic health services should be government provided funded through taxpayer dollars, similar to education, it is referenced as socialism or socialist medicine. If the belief is that health care should be provided privately, then it sits within a more individualistic/behaviorist mindset where people are expected to be self-determined in their pursuit of health and its access. These perspectives sit in stark contrast to each other and harbor very different values about health and whether it is a right or not. Within an individualist tradition, health happens only if you will or can pull yourself up by the bootstraps, do what you need to do to stay healthy and/or afford the costs for your own health. You created your own health circumstance, so you pay for it. It's not my problem, nor is it the governments and I don't want my hard-earned tax dollars to go toward keeping "you" healthy! The only concession made for government-provided health care sit within Medicaid/Medicare programs and as well Veteran Affairs and the passage of the highly contested ACA in 2012. Lobbyists for the two major US political parties officially positioned the narrative from distinct views. The conservative perspective is that a government-run healthcare system will reduce both efficiency and quality of care, as well as compromise the patient-physician relationship and increase waiting times within the healthcare system, as evidenced by government-run healthcare systems around the world (Republicanviews.org, 2016; Grassley, 2009). Liberals, on the other hand, welcome big government involvement in health care and believe they are "fighting to secure universal health care for the American people for generations, and we are proud to be the party that passed Medicare, Medicaid, and the Affordable Care Act".

With the different ideological and political shifts pushed by both the media and the political parties, it can be difficult to establish long-lasting solutions to America's healthcare system's problems. The political divide provides fertile ground for legislative agendas that promote the interest of the position and not its impact on the health outcomes of the consumers. Hence, millions are spent on lobbyists and campaigns to influence the system of care.

Justice in health is not a partisan position, it is a human one. If the healthcare system debate shifts to a human-centered solution, then all considerations would be tailored to solutions that maximize positive outcome for the humans engaged with the system. The care of health would always factor in as its first priority a universal approach to delivering care to all human beings. Universality is fully inclusive of everyone and implies that irrespective of status, ethnicity, gender and identity, all are able to obtain health care. The obvious trajectory to achieve universality in health care would have to involve some level of government, directly or indirectly, as either the providers of health care or as a national health insurer of care, with set fees for service.

While some will argue that this is evidence of big government with an expanded role that infringes on individual rights, it stands to reason that the precedent has already been set with existing federal health and education programs. K-12 education is government funded through tax dollars whether you have children or have children in the K-12 age range. Health care for veterans, the elderly, and those living below the poverty line are covered. Working with the existing infrastructure to mirror these programs does not infringe on it; it actually enhances the scaffolding already in place and the lives of us all. Moreover, for these most important rights that are covered, it has already been determined that the government, given its oversight and responsibility to serve the people, is the only entity that can and should do this.

The government is not a for-profit company; it is a democracy for the people. A for-profit company is operating to make a profit, which puts its very mission in conflict with providing universal care. We are buying care and health, as a commodity…as a business exchange. As a business, revenue is the expected outcome, and not solely the health and well-being of its customers. It can never be. As long as our system of care is subjected to this model, we will continue to have what we have: those who can afford care "buying it" and those who cannot, going without or suffering high mortality and morbidity at embarrassing rates. If neither of those scenarios happen, individuals are subject to run the risk of financial ruin and/or the loss of their home, crippling their ability to ever "buy" health care again.

In this country, the haves and have nots are divided along lines of race, social location, gender and income, making the current structure both inequity and unjust. Health outcomes run along those very clear marginalized lines, and the resulting consequences from the lack of health are also guaranteed along these same lines. Those without health insurance end up getting care when they find themselves in an unavoidable health situation (heart attack, injury, cancer), which generates system costs irrespective of one's ability to pay. Theses costs are absorbed in what is called indigent care so not providing a universal system of care that covers all persons does not stop the need and the responsibility to provide care. It happens anyway. We are better off to plan for how we use those dollars in advance so that it is budgeted in a less reactive way, i.e., less expensive preventative services versus paying for extremely costly tertiary service, lengthy hospital stays, and major medical interventions.

The anticipated outrage in arguments about the cost of providing any form of universal healthcare model can be mitigated by the following facts: that doing nothing costs more; that the current healthcare system is neither cost efficient nor sustainable; and that providing primary health care saves money which is a cost savings offset that will reduce costs. Fighting to keep a system with increasing costs and decreasing access and population health outcomes is not political, it is nonsensical. However, the impetus for rectifying the current structure of health should not be to solely reduce costs; humanely, it is the right thing to do. Nonetheless money is the currency of value, so reform has to lead from the economic argument just presented. The best return on investment for our healthcare system is the upstream investment in public health and prevention. The return on investment is healthy people's healthy lives, reduced costs, increased productivity, longer lives, appropriate use of system services, and decrease in expensive service utilization, service misuse and overuse (of emergency rooms, first responders).

5.4.1   Aligning Health Beliefs, Values, and Actions

Our system of health involves a spectrum of care with competing values and inequitable distribution of resources that primarily are positioned to over respond to sick care and under respond to prevention. Healthcare provider training, resources allocations, and reimbursements mirror this dichotomy. If we are truly in the business of health care, then preservation and the protection of health should be centered and not the restoration of health once it has already been compromised. Addressing health needs with a preventative orientation is beneficial for many reasons that go beyond preventing the onset and progression of disease. Focusing on the upstream and preventative drivers of health would facilitate the system's ability to offset the more costly tertiary interventions by intervening before individuals require more costly care options. Prevention is the central pillar of public health which has already proven a return on investment of 1–4 (Masters et al., 2017).

The United States is overrun by the epidemic of chronic disease and perpetual ineffective response to reducing them. Chronic disease progression can be managed by clinical preventive measures which include intervening before disease develops (primary prevention), diagnosing and treating disease at an early stage (secondary prevention), and managing disease to reduce or halt its course (tertiary prevention) (Levine, 2019). These interventions, when paired with behavioral changes, can significantly lower the incidence of chronic disease, as well as the disability and death that comes with it. Despite the human and economic costs of chronic diseases, we have not made significant headway to prevent or mitigate them and have underutilized population-specific prevention approaches on the frontlines.

Chronic diseases place a significant strain on both patients and the healthcare system. Majority of adults in the United States had at least one chronic disease or condition in 2014, and about half the adult population had multiple diseases (Buttorff et al., 2017). "Chronic diseases, such as heart disease, cancer, chronic lung disease, stroke, Alzheimer's disease, diabetes, osteoarthritis, and chronic kidney disease, are the leading causes of illness, disability, and death in the United States" (Levine, 2019). Rather than preventive care, we have an unbalanced focus on disease, specialty care, and technology. Preventive care lowers the risk of diseases, disabilities, and ; however, millions of Americans do not and cannot receive recommended preventive healthcare services. Children require scheduled vaccinations, routine checkups, and dental visits to ensure healthy development and detect health issues early when they are usually easier to treat. Screenings, dental check-ups, and vaccinations are critical to keeping people of all ages healthy. However, for a variety of reasons, many people experience barriers to obtaining necessary preventive care including cost, the lack of a primary care provider, living too far away from providers, and a lack of awareness about recommended preventive services (Levine, 2019).

Imagine only going to the mechanic when your car is completely broken down: no oil changes, fluid top ups, tire checks, or inspections. Instead, you only deal with the car when it is in complete disrepair and in need of a new engine because you failed to check the oil or a new transmission because you failed to keep the fluids full. The cost of a few quarts of oil and a few bottles of antifreeze are far cheaper than the cost of a new engine or transmission. The same logic can be used to think about health care. It is beyond reasonable to expect then that we have a healthcare system that focuses on the (oil changes and fluids) prevention—than on costly interventions (transmissions and engines) that come with tertiary care. So while we know that this more intense effort will be needed and are necessary to have in place, it should not overshadow all of our other approaches to care. If we can expect this approach at a minimum for a car but why not a human body?

The provocative nature of this analogy does not propose any amelioration of the tertiary system, it does advocate for the refocusing, realignment and integration of system efforts and resources into prevention spaces to achieve greatest health impact for the most amount people to produce the greatest return on our healthcare investment. Those spaces involve access to care but also include access to opportunity and access to innovation. Cross sector policy alignment is essential to support this vision as is evaluation to inform our implementation processes and evidence our outcomes, thus embedding accountability. Fiscal resource allocation will dominate the decision-making about what our system could look like. Proposed would be a system that can deliver an equal if not greater return on investment. In short, a system whose costs do not supersede its impacts and are sustainable at levels comparable to other Organisation for Economic and Co-operative Development (OECD) countries.

5.4.2   Preparing Healthcare Providers

The educational curriculum of many pre- and post-licensure students is dominated by preparation, training, and examination. Students are taught to identify and treat their patient with most of their hands-on training and preparation requiring a significant dose of clinical immersive experiences either in a simulation or OSCELab, on a unit/rotation, during practicum, and as interns. Overwhelming students are being abundantly prepared to care for populations and the health issues they experience. Given the context and focus of our current system and content of licensure examination which heavily tests their knowledge base across similar dimensions, this makes sense.

Population and public health are on the margins of the bulk of coursework, with limited practice focus and less clinical placements throughout all years of the healthcare licensure programs. Health policy exposure in coursework should be a harmonized threat that concurrently is woven through with a health equity lens in all aspects of course work. The disservice that comes from not having robust exposure to the determinants and drivers of health within such a skewed emphasis of physical health and disease is the reinforcement of the status quo which makes change near impossible. As long as we keep preparing our providers to embrace a linear focus and reify a very narrow view of health dominated by the current system's configuration, then we will never produce a sufficient cohort of health providers and future leaders who can even envision a system any differently. Healthcare students should engage with many of the international resolutions such as the United Nations Sustainable Development Goals and endorsed national strategies of Healthy People 2030 as part of their coursework. At a minimum they need awareness, but more importantly they can start to intentionally align their research, science, and practice in contribution to attainment of the goals. Healthcare providers and students have to become influential health policy actors that can inform health policy, respond to health policy, and recommend health policy. At all levels, they must lead the development and analysis of health policies as health experts and mobilize in partnership en masse to lead impactful change. The diversity of expertise by all health professions and health partners is sorely needed at this critical juncture of justice making in health and health equity.

Exposure and immersion in health policy, health equity, preventative practice and public health across every year of training, and significant embedment into examinations, clinical rotations, and internships would create a seismic shift on the future of healthcare system and reimagining of that future. Justice in health dares to imagine that the primary preparation of all healthcare providers occurs within the social determinants of health and social justice paradigm. That means it is evident and infused in every training and educational scenario to the point of complete saturation. This approach would serve to insulate any preparation so that the social determinants of health and social justice does not become the orientation of a few but becomes the overwhelming view of many and eventually the default aspiration of what health must be. The present approach would instead be re-ordered to feed into one's unique health situation with the fullest awareness and consideration of the context, experiences, and conditions surrounding the patient's health. The dots of that patient's overall health and well-being would be connected so that a holistic picture and holistic solution can be generated. We would meet the patient where they are and better positioned to react more appropriately across primary and secondary lines of the patient or client's health context. With this information, providers are then able to thoroughly vet and exhaust efforts to mitigate barriers to health. Approaching patients' determinants upfront and as part of their care becomes the first resort and no longer the last. Students become deeply engaged with the entire human condition versus an episode of it. They would be better equipped to make connections with the determinants of health and health outcomes.

Infusing more health innovation into education with protected space for social entrepreneurism would further advance healthcare education and the development of solutions. Inclusive health pedagogy taught inside and outside of traditional health disciplines opens up the possibility for non-siloed education that builds a community of transdisciplinary learners who are passionate about health and can work together to co-create equitable health solutions. Creating opportunities for innovative discovery and context-based solutions would deepen and evolve students' critical awareness, unleashing untapped potential that would benefit us all. We would ensure that all students have the capacity and tools to become the next generation of healthcare leaders who can imagine and advocate for policy and structural changes that support human thriving and flourishing. Students would be exposed to a wider cadre of skills and expertise that allow them to work more collaboratively in a transdisciplinary manner across settings and in non-traditional teams. This creates cohorts of health justice practitioners and leaders trained to facilitate transformative change in the lives and health of their communities and not sustain health disparities and inequities by failing to act on root causes and solutions.

Being deeply immersed as thought and action partners in addressing societal issues that lead to poor health outcomes will have become the new norm and practice expectation with altruistic benefits becoming more appealing than the financial ones. Taking a multi-faceted approach with a ferocious commitment to ameliorating root causes of health disparities is the impact and mission of health "care" at the most primal of levels. Our inaction to courageously change the current direction of the existing system has caused a tremendous amount of burden to our healthcare system, its capacity, and disproportionate suffering of disparate populations. Even more troubling is the further erosion of trust that occurs by the inconsistency of our commitment to do no harm while inadvertently doing the complete opposite.

Historically, we are reminded that health care in the United States has had a track record of inhumane abuses and medical exploitation of minoritized populations which have been documented over the years and has broken trust. Restoring trust of the community will need to begin with building relationships and reestablishing a new social health contract as a system and as providers. Justice in health prepares students to proactively engage with the community where they are—where they live, work, and play (in their homes, neighborhoods, churches, community gathering spaces). This is the starting point for rebuilding trust and healing and where health really happens. Overtime, one can foresee communities that are emboldened with the support of healthcare providers to define health needs and optimize the potential to thrive fostered by a health infrastructure which makes it possible.

For all providers, the unique non-medical history and context of the individual should be the first step in gathering "health" history. Asking individuals questions about their presenting state only superficially capture the history of a very narrow health view. What it does not capture are the individuals' circumstances, the determinants of their health, the structural barriers to achieving health, and everything else in between. These "other" dimensions of health show up and present as disease and in many cases as trauma.

5.5 Trauma-Informed Approaches

Trauma is the exposure to harmful and negative sequelae such as violence, abuse, neglect, loss, war, and other intensive stressors and events that deeply impact emotional, social, physical, and spiritual well-being (SAMHSA, 2014). Because it is a known risk factor to substance use, physical illness, and mental and behavioral health challenges and presents itself across sectors and situations, it cannot be left unaddressed. Trauma is widespread and far-reaching with exposures touching the lives of most Americans. As a known root cause of many presenting conditions, trauma is best assumed given its prevalence in the population and its impacts. According to the US Government Substance Abuse and Mental Health Services Administration (2014), "people with traumatic experiences, however, do not show up only in behavioral health systems. Responses to these experiences often manifest in behaviors or conditions that result in involvement with the child welfare and the criminal and juvenile justice system or in difficulties in the education, employment or primary care system." p. 5. The connection to trauma and adverse health effects has been studied intensively by the adverse childhood experiences (ACE) study revealing lower life expectancy, brain dysregulation, and diminished health outcomes (National Council for Behavioral Health, 2022). It has been found to increase risk of serious health problems "including chronic lung, heart, and livers disease as well as depression, sexually transmitted disease, tobacco, alcohol and illicit drug use throughout life" (Meschner & Maul, 2016).

Although trauma exposure transcends gender, race, and identity, it does affect the most vulnerable of populations disproportionately. Almost half of youth experience at least one traumatic event and close to 2/3 of adults have reported at least one exposure (National Council for Behavioral Health). However, "individuals who identify as black, Hispanic, multiracial, with incomes of less than 15,000 a year and are unemployed" (National Council for Behavioral Health, p. 3) are affected at higher rates. Aggregate populations within these most vulnerable groups such as LGBTQIA and urban populations have shown higher rates of trauma exposure as well (National Council for Behavioral Health). Many of these populations and those most vulnerable among them experience individual and cumulative trauma as a result of their historical and ongoing exposures.

People and communities at risk experience harsh traumatic conditions that alter the trajectory of their lives profoundly and significantly. Historic and cumulative trauma experienced by many communities, particularly communities of color, have generational implications. To treat an individual is to also treat the community and recognize how trauma is impacting their ability to both thrive and flourish. Trauma induces physical and psychological manifestations that show up as ailments (headaches, stomach pains, sleep disorders), unhealthy behaviors (substance use, smoking), negative health consequences (chronic disease, gastrointestinal disorders, anxiety, depression), and adverse childhood exposure (ACES). While the presenting issue is the obvious starting point, using a more holistic treatment approach considers trauma and/or trauma exposure as a possible root cause.

Healthcare providers and systems of care must understand and recognize the impacts of trauma and use trauma-informed approaches in the delivery of care to not retraumatize individuals, families, and communities. This approach acknowledges "the need to understand a patient's life experiences in order to deliver effective care and has the potential to improve patient engagement, treatment adherence, health outcome and provider and staff wellness" (Meschner & Maul, 2016, p. 1). It is a priority approach that needs to be embedded at all system access points knowing the prevalence of trauma and the likelihood of encountering someone exposed to trauma at any point of care and across the lifespan. The US Government Substance Abuse and Mental Health Services Administration (SAMSHA) has proposed a working framework for designing a trauma-informed system of care that is responsive and promotes healing. Within this framework are four assumptions, six principles, and ten implementation domains.

5.5.1 The Four Assumptions of Trauma (SAMHSA, 2014, p. 9)

Assumption 1: Realization: All individuals at all levels of the organization have a realization of trauma and understand its effects at the individual, family, and community level. They understand how the context of trauma intersects with and shapes experiences and behaviors with an interrelatedness across sectors.

Assumption 2: Recognition: Of the signs and symptoms of trauma.

Assumption 3: Respond: The organization and its structures broadly assume trauma exposure and apply a trauma-informed approach that is evident in its mission, policies, practices, programs, and culture. The organization provides a physical and psychologically safe environment and invest resources (training, budget, mentoring) to uphold these practices.

Assumption 4: Resist: Is the organizations' intention to resist re-victimization of victims in their operations and approaches to care.

5.5.2 The Six Principles of Trauma-Informed Care (SAMHSA, 2014, p. 10)

1. Safety-Feelings of physical and psychological safety in settings and interactions.
2. Trustworthiness and Transparency-Organizational operation and decisions are conducted with transparency toward building and maintaining trust.
3. Peer Support-Key to establishing safety, hope, building trust, promoting recovery, and healing.
4. Collaboration and Mutuality-Meaningful partnership and sharing of power.
5. Empowerment, Voice, and Choice-Belief in resilience and understands the need to foster empowerment and cultivating self-advocacy, facilitating choice, and goal-setting.
6. Cultural, Historical, and Gender Issues-Moves past cultural stereotypes and biases in structures, accessibility, and values.

The provider oriented within a justice-in-health lens must examine and weigh multiple intersecting layers which requires a practice skill set that explores the situatedness of the individual. Patient histories can no longer heavily rely on the biological to the exclusion of ecological and the contextual. While integrating this level of comprehensiveness to any patient/client encounter will require the investment of more time by the healthcare provider, the client will benefit from receiving care that is better informed by the totality of factors that are contributing to their health situation. Moreover, it exposes the barriers to the individual's ability to achieve health and subsequently creates an opportunity to connect the individual with the resources to overcome these barriers. Anything less than this will continue to result in persistent use and mismatch of use of the healthcare system. When providers and healthcare systems move toward instilling a trauma-informed system of care, resilience factors that build hope and strengthen the individual and their community from adverse situations are critical components for inclusion (National Council for Behavioral Health).

To deepen the engagement between healthcare providers and their clients creates the need for an intensified focus on appreciative inquiry, cultural humility, antiracism, and trauma-informed care. Diversity, equity, and inclusion also have to be a curriculum thread woven through all pre-licensure training in an immersive way. Our intention must be to ensure that engagement with traumatized communities is neither re-traumatizing nor re-victimizing.

5.6 Proposition

While there are many critical areas examined through the lens of Justice in Health, many remain unexplored. It would take an extensive amount of investigation and research to unpack all of the nuances and weeds clogging up our system of care. However, that does not mean the system itself cannot be reimagined in a systematic and concrete way based on what is known.

Considering much of the discourse and dialogue that has occurred in this and previous chapters, the following recommendations for rebuilding a more equitable, just, and sovereign system of health must involve these fundamental steps.

A National Dialogue: One of the many opportunities that COVID created has been the opportunity for dialogue around health disparities due to the unavoidable spotlight of the inequitable impacts of COVID on vulnerable populations. While the dialogue was triggered by COVID's accelerated proliferation in our society and its simultaneously paralyzing effects on the economy, health system, education, and families, it was not structured or coordinated. Essentially that and most dialogue around our system has also mirrored this same approach: fractured, unplanned, and not toward any real coordinated strategy for moving forward. A nationally commissioned dialogue with an intentional mandate of leading the charge toward envisioning a new model for health care is an important step to truly changing the current system. What it looks like, how long it occurs, and who are the key stakeholders to be involved can be determined by an appointed national dialogue committee charged with leading the design and development of the dialogue process. Part of the process will involve mass mobilization of stakeholders from various sectors, designating strategic areas of focus for the dialogue process (implementation strategy, budget strategy, healthcare professional strategy, resources, and capacity strategy), and the creation of the overarching dialogue implementation strategy and development of recommendations for next steps based on the findings from the processes.

A National Dialogue Process: The initiation of a national dialogue process with the goal of defining and reimagining health and our system of health in the United States. This process should not be developed exclusively by healthcare professionals. Instead, it should be constructed by design thinking experts, community members, and those on the front lines of the health system (Note: health system is defined within a Justice in Health orientation and includes the determinants of health). The process should be clearly formulated and outlined with clear objectives, implementation plan, expected outcomes, and impact areas, timelines with clear philosophical principles about health. Moreover, the process must involve input from each State and have engagement that is representative of the US population in terms of gender, ethnicity, age, and geographical location. Both the process and oversight of the process must be funded by the government or a multistakeholder consortium from end to end. Accountability is woven into the process through establishment mechanisms for evaluation, data collection, and analysis that produce outcomes to inform a potential structure. While many of the investments in dismantling the current system must be made to our basic principles, all efforts for rethinking what health and subsequently health care in this country can be are long overdue and necessary.

*A **National 'Health as Humanity' Strategy:*** Both the national dialogue and the dialogue process should support and orbit a central theme. Based on what has been discussed through a justice-in-health approach, the goal of health sovereignty for individuals, community, and society is fueled by the understanding of health not simply as a right but as a strategy for humanity must prevail. Health as a strategy for humanity strikes the chord that to be healthy is to be in the fullness of ones' humanity and hence is not separate from, but a part of, humanness. While it might be assumed that this is fundamental to the belief in our existing system of health, the inability or decision not to implement a system where health is a human right provides evidences to the contrary. Should the country and national truly live the values of health as a human right, then the system of health must reflect this belief. Its current focus and configuration do not. What we witness is a system of inequity, injustice, and inhumanity for those who are fortunate to access it.

Health as humanity structurally reflects and reconciles that having health is essential to our existence and inherent right as humans. Without health, our humanity will neither thrive nor can it flourish so our health system's structural alignment with this core mission has to become a built-in imperative. Building in this imperative systemically requires unfettered access across the spectrum of health care and the re-centering or policies, practices, and procedures that can facilitate this understanding.

Consider Creating a System Without Walls: encompasses a reimagined system which demonstrates the resetting of our healthcare values based on *Justice in Health* philosophies. Aligned with such a design are the delivery and execution of health, health services, and access to those services with justice and equity. The system of health no longer is confined to being actualized within one certain space and only by a limited body of health brokers. Instead, the system health transcends the confinement of walled structures to engage in community spaces, neighborhood spaces, schools, and homes. A system without walls approach builds a health orientation that fosters unencumbered access at multiple entry points and using methods that enhance access.

The health system without walls is not a static entity that people go to—it transcends, becomes a part of existing all of our health and health-related structures, and is also intentionally infused into populations and programs by design. It is proactively responsive to human lives in ways that are nimble and adaptable. What must be a part of any system without walls is the embodiment of a health and health equity in all policies approach with people-centered care policies. Health and health equity in all policies espouses exactly what it says; that health should be woven in all policies with health understood more broadly to include the social determinants. Inclusion of a more expansive vision of health into all policies means that transportation, housing, environment, and economic policies, for example, are crafted to intentionally embed the optimization of human health. Such policies become human centered when they leverage assets and foster autonomy and resilience. They further serve to unify policy intent around a common mandate of health which could mediate unintended consequences of the policies. A common health mandate helps to align policies with each other and form cohesive integration of any intersecting policy mandates which makes them complementary to each other and to building the capacity for health in individuals, communities, and society. Alignment mitigates policy contradictions between policies and positions government structures with an inherent coordinated public health approach.

Practice Competencies: Expanded competencies would have to be required of providers to meet this re-envisioned version of our health system and its emergent approaches. Training and education must mirror the vision by adopting transdisciplinary partnerships that bring healthcare disciplines and non-healthcare disciplines together to incubate and co-create solutions. New and renewed curricula that examine race, history, trauma, and the requiring of humanity-based skills and competencies (diversity, equity, inclusion, cultural humility, mindfulness, appreciative inquiry) should be necessary and fundamental learning for all professions. Health disciplines need to expand their curriculum to focus on a more futuristic vision of health care, where team science and engagement are shared outside of discipline tracts. It must also be where entrepreneurship, civic engagement, and social innovation are core curriculum elements and healthcare providers are adaptable providers across settings and spaces where people live, work, and play.

The healthcare provider of a reimagined system such as the one being proposed works alongside environmental engineers, artists, city planners, political scientists, and business administrators to integrate and translate expert health knowledge into holistic health solutions. They are employable in multiple sectors in capacities that go beyond traditional health sector positions and can advise, lead, and implement health at various levels of government, community, and individual levels as the dot connectors, innovators, and threaders of health.

5.7 Reflective Questions and Considerations

1. How can trauma-informed approaches be integrated in your practice/ organizations?
2. What could a reimagined healthcare system look like in the United States? What steps need to occur to make it happen?
3. What would you propose as an action step to create a system without walls?

References

ABC News. (n.d.-a). *Why the US spends more on health care than other countries, but doesn't fare better: Study*. ABC News. Retrieved February 28, 2022, from https://abcnews.go.com/Health/us-spends-health-care-countries-fare-study/story?id=53710650

Archer, D. (2019). Health care costs continue to rise faster than inflation. Dec 11, 2019. Retrieved Nov 2, 2022 from: https://abcnews.go.com/Health/us-spends-health-care-countries-fare-study/story?id=53710650.

American Medical Association. Retrieved April 2, 2022 from Value-based Patient-Centered Care | American Medical Association (ama-assn.org).

Blumenthal, D., Miller, M. E., & Gustafsson, L. (2021, October 1). The U.S. can lower drug prices without sacrificing innovation. *Harvard Business Review*. https://hbr.org/2021/10/the-u-s-can-lower-drug-prices-without-sacrificing-innovation

Butkus, R., Rapp, K., Cooney, T., & Engel, L. (2020). *Addressing social determinants to improve patient care and promote health equity: An American College of Physicians Position Paper*. Annuals of Internal Medicine. Supplement: Vision for U.S. Health Care, 21 January 2020, Retrieved from: https://www.acpjournals.org/doi/full/10.7326/M19-2410

Buttorff, C., Ruder, T., & Bauman, M. (2017). *Multiple chronic conditions in the United States*. RAND Corporation. https://www.rand.org/pubs/tools/TL221.html

Crenshawe, K. (1991, July). Mapping the margins: Intersectionality, identity politics, and violence against women of color. *Stanford Law Review, 43*(6), 1241–1299. https://doi.org/10.2307/1229039

Dec 13, P. U. P. & 2017. (2017, December 13). Living in an immigrant family in America: How fear and toxic stress are affecting daily life, well-being, & health. *KFF*. https://www.kff.org/racial-equity-and-health-policy/issue-brief/living-in-an-immigrant-family-in-america-how-fear-and-toxic-stress-are-affecting-daily-life-well-being-health/

Democratic View on Health Care | Republican Views. (2014, October 20). https://www.republican-views.org/democratic-view-on-health-care/

De Lew, N., Greenberg, G., & Kinchen, K. (1992). A layman's guide to the US health care system. *Health Care Financing Review, 14*(1), 151.

Eklund, J. H., Holmström, I. K., Kumlin, T., Kaminsky, E., Skoglund, K., Höglander, J., ... & Meranius, M. S. (2019). "Same same or different?" A review of reviews of person-centered and patient-centered care. *Patient Education and Counseling, 102*(1), 3–11.

Government of Canada. (2019). *Canada's health system*. Retrieved July 10, 2022 from: https://www.canada.ca/en/health-canada/services/health-care-system/reports-publications/health-care-system/canada.html#a8

Government of the United States. (2022, March 2). Full transcript of Biden's State of the Union address. *The New York Times*. https://www.nytimes.com/2022/03/01/us/politics/biden-sotu-transcript.html

Grassley, C. (2009). Health care reform—A republican view. *New England Journal of Medicine, 361*(25), 2397–2399. https://doi.org/10.1056/NEJMp0911111

Hansson, E., Ekman, I., Swedberg, K., Wolf, A., Dudas, K., Ehlers, L., & Olsson, L. E. (2016). Person-centred care for patients with chronic heart failure—A cost-utility analysis. *European Journal of Cardiovascular Nursing, 15*, 276–284.

Health Care. (n.d.). *Democrats*. Retrieved February 28, 2022, from https://democrats.org/where-we-stand/the-issues/health-care/

Lazar, L., & Davenport, L. (2018). Barriers to health care access for low income families: A review of literature. *Journal of Community Health Nursing, 35*(1), 28–37. https://doi.org/10.1080/07370016.2018.1404832

Levine, S. (2019). Health care industry insights: Why the use of preventive services is still low. *Preventing Chronic Disease, 16*. https://doi.org/10.5888/pcd16.180625

Martin, D., Miller, A., Quesnel-Vallée, A., Caron, N., Vissandjée, B., & Marchildon, G. (2018). Canada's universal health system: Achieving its potential. *The Lancet, 391*, 1718–1735. https://doi.org/10.1016/S0140-6736(18)30181-8

Masters, R., Anwar, E., Collins, B., Cookson, R., & Capewell, S. (2017, August). Return on investment of public health interventions: A systematic review. *Journal of Epidemiology and Community Health, 71*(8), 827–834. https://doi.org/10.1136/jech-2016-208141. Epub 2017 Mar 29. PMID: 28356325; PMCID: PMC5537512.

Meschner, C., & Maul, A. (2016). *Key ingredient for successful trauma-informed care implementation*. Center for Health Care Strategies.

National Council for Behavioral Health. (2022). *Trauma-informed primary care: Fostering resilience and recovery. A change package for advancing trauma-informed primary care*. National Council for Behavioral Health.

Nomura, H., & Nakayama, T. (2005). The Japanese healthcare system. *BMJ: British Medical Journal, 331*(7518), 648–649.

Palfreman, J., & Reid, T. R. (2008). *Sick around the World*. Boston, MA: WGBH Educational Foundation, PBS Home Video: United States of America.

Papanicolas, I., Woskie, L., and Jha, A. (2018). Health Care Spending in the United States and Other High-Income Countries," *Journal of the American Medical Association, 319*(10), 1024–39. https://doi.org/10.26099/ts8g-dj28

Peter G Foundation (2019). Why are prescription drug prices rising and how do they affect the US fiscal outlook? Retrieved Nov 2, 2022from: https://www.pgpf.org/blog/2019/11/why-are-prescription-drug-prices-rising-and-how-do-they-affect-the-us-fiscaloutlook#:~:text=The%20Total%20Cost%20of%20Prescription%20Drugs%20Is%20Projected,in%202007%20to%20%241%2C025%20per%20capita%20in%202017.

Pirhonen, L., Hansson Olofsson, E., Fors, A., Ekman, I., & Bolin, K. (2017). Effects of person-centred care on health outcomes—A randomized controlled trial in patients with acute coronary syndrome. *Health Policy, 121*(2), 169–179, ISSN 0168-8510. https://doi.org/10.1016/j.healthpol.2016.12.003

Republican Views on Health Care | Republican Views. (2014, November 26). https://www.republicanviews.org/republican-views-on-health-care/

Retired health care workers answer the call for help amid COVID-19 pandemic. (2020, March 17). *Coronavirus*. https://www.ctvnews.ca/health/coronavirus/retired-health-care-workers-answer-the-call-for-help-amid-covid-19-pandemic-1.4857581

Rosso, R. J. (2021). *U.S. Health care coverage and spending*. 3.

SAMHSA. (2014). Retrieved April 16, 2021 from https://ncsacw.acf.hhs.gov/userfiles/files/SAMHSA_Trauma.pdf

Scutti, S. (2019, January 23). *Big Pharma spends record millions on lobbying amid pressure to lower drug prices*. CNN. https://www.cnn.com/2019/01/23/health/phrma-lobbying-costs-bn/index.html

Sick Around The World. (n.d.). *Frontline*. Retrieved March 13, 2022, from https://www.pbs.org/wgbh/frontline/film/sickaroundtheworld/

United States Government. The Whitehouse (2022) State of the union addresss March 1 (2022) Retrieved Nov 2, 2022 from: https://www.whitehouse.gov/state-ofthe-union-2022/

U.S. Physician Shortage Growing. (n.d.). *AAMC*. Retrieved March 7, 2022, from https://www.aamc.org/news-insights/us-physician-shortage-growing

Weatherby Blog. (2021). *Physician salary report 2021: Doctor's compensation steady.* Published May 26, 2021. Accessed 13 Mar 2022. https://weatherbyhealthcare.com/blog/annual-physician-salary-report

What are the recent and forecasted trends in prescription drug spending? (n.d.). *Peterson-KFF health system tracker*. Retrieved March 6, 2022, from https://www.healthsystemtracker.org/chart-collection/recent-forecasted-trends-prescription-drug-spending/

Weatherby Healthcare (2021). Physician salary report 2021, Compensation steady despite COVID-19 Retreived Nov 2, 2022 from: https://weatherbyhealthcare.com/blog/annual-physician-salary-report-2021

Wilcox, L. (2021). Physician Salary Report 2021: *Compensation Steady Despite COVID-19.* Weatherby Healthcare. https://weatherbyhealthcare.com/blog/annual-physician-salary-report

Wu, T.-Y., Majeed, A., & Kuo, K. N. (2010). An overview of the healthcare system in Taiwan. *London Journal of Primary Care, 3*(2), 115–119.

Chapter 6
Leading Through Just Action

This chapter introduces readers to community engagement and partnerships as facilitators to rebuilding and co-creating a system of care. Understanding community partnership and their importance are discussed. Examining practice partnerships and best practice approaches for engaging with the community to meet their health needs where they are is a central component of this chapter. The chapter draws on community engagement and partnership exemplars from the field that have been used to demonstrate how communities can mobilize and transform health. It also discusses the use and power of platforms such as media for advocacy and use of data as tools for change. The chapter serves to help health providers, health researchers, and health educators consider non-traditional approaches to creatively find ways to exchange knowledge, skills, and expertise needed to reform and redress health disparities. It is a chapter to remind healthcare providers to act effectively to create and influence equitable health solutions.

6.1 Community Engagement: So What and Who Cares?

Community engagement has gained increasing visibility in educational programs particularly in practice and research. The term has been used loosely to describe a broad spectrum of community-connected activities from service learning, internships, community immersion experiences, community collaboration events, community located activities, and research partnerships with community members. It is erroneously referenced when making the most minimal of touchpoints with a community as representative of community engagement. While the term has been used out of context and in misalignment with what true community engagement is and should be, its significance cannot be overstated. Fully actualized community engagement is the most essential requirement in the attainment of just and equitable health. Recognizing its value and power to bring action when properly harnessed is mission critical to the reimagining and recalibrating of our system of health. As with the examination of the terminology and contextualization of health, a similar approach to unpacking community engagement is needed as a starting point to inform all else. We will also explore community engagement across the spectrum as a way of knowing, as a way of being, and as a way of doing.

C. Burnett, *Justice in Health*, https://doi.org/10.1007/978-3-031-18504-5_6

6.2   Community Engagement as a Way of Knowing

Community engagement is transformative and fundamental to mobilizing meaningful change in our healthcare system. Increasingly it has become an instrument of civic democracy and innovation that promotes good citizenship and social responsibility by individuals, organizations, and institutions. It describes collaboration and partnerships with community for the benefit of community that is rooted in reciprocity, trust, and equity. There is a social currency that comes with community engagement where ideas, values, expertise, and vision are equitably exchanged to yield solutions. The ability of community engagement to inform a range of issues and the recognition of its benefit has increased the visibility and usage of community engagement.

Health disparities, social justice, and social innovation are some of the many drivers of community engagement influencing its uptake and more recently the urgency for increasing its use. Institutions of Higher Education in particular have incubated community engagement through community-engaged scholarship, student community-based internships, practicums and service learning as a pillar of student learning, student success, and student training. Not only have these institutions used community engagement as one of its core approaches across these experiential areas, they are quite motivated to do so. One institutional motivation that is highly sought after by Institutions of Higher Education in the United States is the Carnegie Foundation for the Advancement of Teaching Community Engagement Elective Classification (https://carnegieelectiveclassifications.org/the-elective-classification-for-community-engagement-2/). This elective classification is bestowed for a 6-year time frame to an institution reflecting its commitment to community engagement as reflected achievement of key milestones in the areas of community-engaged scholarship, civic engagement, and service-learning activities of faculty, staff, and students.

The Carnegie Foundation for the Advancement of Teaching defines community engagement as "the collaboration between institutions of higher education and their larger communities (local, regional/state, national, global) for the mutually beneficial creation and exchange of knowledge and resources in a context of partnership and reciprocity" (2022, p. 1). They go further to state the purpose of community engagement is "the partnership (of knowledge and resources) between colleges and universities and the public and private sectors to enrich scholarship, research, and creative activity; enhance curriculum, teaching, and learning; prepare educated, engaged citizens; strengthen democratic values and civic responsibility; address critical societal issues; and contribute to the public good" (2022, p. 2).

Like Carnegie, the Association of Public and Land-grant Universities also provides leadership and guidance in community engagement activities to academic institutions through its Commission on Economic and Community Engagement (https://www.aplu.org/our-work/5-archived-projects/economic-development-and-community-engagement/). This Commission offers awards, designations, and the important work of convening leadership from institutions toward the goal of focusing "on imagining and then realizing a shared vision for healthier and more engaged citizens, thriving economies, and other outcomes that lead to a better tomorrow." They share resources that include blueprints and frameworks and lift up national university exemplars of community engagement.

Beyond formal designation, accolades, and in some cases accreditation requirements, institutions have found that community engagement provides enriching opportunities to extend its reach and impact. Student success in Institutions of Higher Education is influenced by high impact practices of experiential learning (Bradberry & De Maio, 2019; Roberts, 2018) while community-engaged research provides the avenue for intellectualism and activism which are high priority traits of Generation Xers and Millennials (Lynch-Alexander, 2017). With community engagement's heightened profile as a high-impact practice, accelerated and far-reaching expansion is increasingly encouraged. Such fevered progress should be viewed with cautious optimism given the potential for institutions and its actors to misstep, fracturing relationships, trust, and opportunities for further engagement. Without the proper infrastructure, knowledge, and preparation to do community-engaged work, the chance of missteps, irrespective of intention, are a real possibility and expected. To be in relation with the community carries an enormous amount of responsibility that should be respected and reflected in all facets of the institutions work that extends into the community.

Strum et al. (2011) examine the relational aspects of community engagement within the academic institution, proposing that its practices, goals, and experiences are interdependent. Using an architectural construct based on the belief in full participation of all, they propose that "—what and who is valued, how decisions are made, which interests matter, who gets to participate, how work is organized, how problems are addressed—cuts across diversity, public scholarship, and student success work, and currently poses barriers to all" (Strum et al., 2011, p. 5). They purport that integration of knowledge, diversity, and resources are essential to the legitimacy, efficacy, and sustainability of community-engaged work as it allows for more effective connection with each other and the values and practices of the institution.

Community-engaged scholarship tends to attract scholars who reflect the diversity of the community they wish to engage with. However, experiences of epistemic exclusion frequently encountered by faculty of color and women impede the opportunity for community-engaged scholarship and create barriers to success. Settles et al. (2022) refer to epistemic exclusion as "the devaluation of marginalized scholars and scholarship that falls outside of a field's disciplinary center, asserting that they do not contribute meaningfully to knowledge production" (p. 33). It is "a form of scholarly delegitimization rooted in disciplinary biases about what types of research are valued as well as social identity-based biases against individuals from marginalized groups" (Settles et al., 2022, p. 32). Those engaged in community-engaged scholarship have the responsibility of legitimizing their work to meet expected performance outcomes that might work for traditional approaches but are much harder to achieve in community-engaged work. For example, community engagement requires the building and sustaining of meaningful relationships with the community. This requires an enormous amount of committed time and seemingly invisible work that interfere with other requirements of "success." Requirements of success in Institutions of Higher Education could be annual publications and grants. While those outcomes are reasonable expectations of any scholar, for those engaged in community-engaged scholarship, relationship-building is a necessary part of the process that will eventually lead to expected outcomes of scholarship products. However, the upfront investment of time in the establishment of the relationship and involvement of the community can slow down the scholarship productivity which might carry negative career consequences in the future. Encouraging the prioritization of community-engaged efforts must come with the structural legitimization of community-engaged scholarship. This can happen by auditing discrediting policies and practices that are not conducive to supporting community-engaged scholarship. It will also require academia at large to do a deeper exploration of itself starting with interrogating promotion and tenure requirements (values of the majority are imposed on the minority as to what "counts"), amount of research funding (where the total dollar amount of research grant received is valued based on the project and not the amount), journal publication opportunities (to publish work about minoritized populations generated from community-engaged scholarship) which are less likely available in mainstreamed journals, and methods used to do community-engaged/social justice work as viewed as inferior (Settles et al., 2019). Justice in health demands the alignment of expectation with the intention to successfully do community-engaged work by removing visible and invisible structural impediments.

The recent societal shifts fueled by racial injustice, the pandemic, and social and political protests have only heightened the rally cry for more community-engaged work to address social justice and inequity. Its rise in prominence as a mechanism for achieving social good comes with cautious optimism until there is a shift in ensuring the internal fidelity that must be in place to do this work well. Community engagement activities do bring a wealth of opportunity to institutions and when enacted properly, can be highly beneficial to the community and the institution. Supporting those who do the work and protecting the community involved in the work is part of community engagement. Be mindful that community engagement can become invasive in its consumption of community spaces, resources, and knowledge and selfishly produce one directional benefit that breaches trust. While we have to be careful to engage with a community with non-maleficence (to do no harm), we also must be expected to practice with the expectation of beneficence, to do good and have the ability to hold both simultaneously. As such, considering community engagement as a tool for good citizenship carries the responsibility of understanding and being a good citizen and what is required to achieve good citizenship.

6.3 Community Engagement as a Tool for Good Citizenship

The importance of community engagement as a tool for good citizenship by institutions is contextualized within the history of the community, the history of the institution, and the history of the institution in relation to the community. Institutions of Higher Education have historically had tenuous and strained relationships with their communities frequently referred to as "a town and gown" relationship. Often, they are among the largest economic engines of the community which has not brought the return to the community as the community would have liked or that they value. In actuality, it has been perceived to cost the community assets, land, created cascading gentrification, and mistreatment/exploitation. Innovation and experimentation are at the forefront of universities-stained history of abuses of its community members. Eugenics, medical experimentation without consent, racial segregation of its education and treatment services, and discriminatory practices are just some of the many ways that these institutions have engaged with the community causing irreparable harm, deep distrust, and alienation.

Disparity in communities with Institutions of Higher Education remains high, even though it is home to many world-class scholars. Economic inequity is prolific in university communities, yet the universities have large operating budgets and assets that eclipse the GDP of small countries. Institutions of Higher Education have state-of-the-art medical services, yet its very own residents cannot access nor afford its care. They are a beacon of education, incubator of ideas, and innovation yet the surrounding public-school systems are depleted and in some areas experience high dropout rates and low achievement scores. As anchor institutions of the community, being a good community citizen is essential but what does that actually mean—what constitutes good citizenship, what is the role and responsibilities of good citizenship?

6.3.1 Understanding the Role and Responsibility of Good Citizenship

Being a good citizen is more actionable than aspirational. Anchor institutions that convey their citizenship in missions and values and their actions as a collective are the demonstration of good citizenship. Gaps perceived by the community or misalignment between the words and actions of the institution are incongruent with good citizenship. More practically, it is akin to behaving badly while proclaiming to be a good person. While the case may very well be that you are a good person, your behaviors say otherwise and help lead others to the belief (real or perceived) that you are not a good person. Similar rules apply with institutions. Stating that you are good, equitable, inclusive, and committed to the greater community in aspirational statements does not assume that you are, especially if the historical and persistent actions are contrary.

Nothing erodes institutional credibility faster and more irreparably than broken trust. Without trust, you cannot build meaningful community relationships or effectively engage in community work. The role of the institution in establishing itself as a good citizen is earning, keeping, and restoring trust with the community. All engagement efforts must embrace trust-building and trust-sustaining actions starting with the acknowledgment of historical acts of abuse or misuse of trust, rectifying past areas of trust failure, providing transparency in actions and intentions, and being consistent in our acts and actions of trust. The actors who are the carriers and actors of the institution's mission also must be trustworthy. Mayne and Geibel (2018) balance the responsibility to be good between the institution's performance and its actors which creates an "inter component congruence" whereas both the institution and its citizens are good.

The hallmark of good citizenship is being trustworthy, not causing harm and doing good. Well-intended community engagement efforts and actors can be harmful.

Community-engagement efforts carry an enormous amount of social responsibility and an inherent assumption of doing good which makes it even more important to ensure the safety of the community in our practices. Operating within the fullest awareness of the historical context, upfront involvement of community expertise and integration of the culture of the community can build in protections for the community which honor its members. The expectation from a justice-in-health position is that both protective and accountability measures are instilled from the initiation of all community activities through until the end. How this occurs is determined and informed by the community. The role and responsibility of the institution is to engage in brave listening and just action to ensure that they engage with true benevolence.

6.4 Community Engagement as Ways of Being

Institutions of Higher Education are structurally complex, largely bureaucratic entities that walk a fine line between that of a large-sized business and as a public-serving institution. Balancing these potentially conflicting mandates create institutional structures and practices that affect how institutions engage with the community. Both missions can happen in healthy synergy with the community when examined with the intention for that to occur. All aspects of institutional practices would need to be reviewed considering barriers and facilitators to community engagement. Areas that warrant particular attention:

Acknowledgment and Reconciliation of History Institutions and communities have history and to engage with the community you must be knowledgeable of that history, consider the impact of that history has on the work you are embarking on, and acknowledge the respective role that the institution plays and continues to play in that history. Know the stories of the history and how they continue to shape the outcomes for the community and the relationships with the community. Start to explore how the institution can rectify its history with the community and implement reconciliatory remedies that are important to the community. Recognize that historical patterns persist because unexamined institutional practice, policies, and procedures continue that erode community trust. The history of mistrust in healthcare providers goes as far back to exploitation and brutalization of Black bodies in slavery and persisted in various forms into recent generations (as discussed in previous chapters). Human experimentation without consent, forced sterilization, segregation of health services by race, and the ongoing racial differences in the quality of health care and health outcomes is the root of the mistrust. Overcoming this history requires, first, acknowledgment followed by radical changes in practices, structures, and preparation of healthcare providers that build and sustain trust. Healthy community engagement will not happen until this occurs. Therefore, build in new practices and structures that support health community engagement and foster a return on the trust of the community. One example of trust is through truth telling such as *Acknowledgment of Country* or *Land Acknowledgment* that respectfully recognizes and names the Indigenous people and their lands that has been colonized and that which institutions and settlers continue to occupy.

Equitable Policies/Procedures   Structures operate within all institutions either mitigating or perpetuating inequities which impede the institutions capacity for benevolent and good community engagement. Institutions should institutionalize structural justice as an operational and moral imperative. According to Burnett et al. (2018), structural justice acknowledges the oppressive and re-victimizing inherent nature of structures as unacceptable and requires purposeful rectification. It demands that primacy and privilege be extended to the most vulnerable, through sustainable structural processes that attend to equity, power, and human dignity (p. 63). Setting up a foundation of structural justice will accomplish much but importantly builds into the system structures that buffer the vulnerability of the most vulnerable and leads the institution away from re-victimizing practices by design to equitable policies and procedures. Having equity structurally embedded will not eliminate harmful practices; however it is one of many needed safeguards that bring institutions closer to this goal. How community work is done will require the support of institutional policies and procedures that ensure it is done equitably and uses best practice approaches. Aspects where institutional policies intersect with community-engaged work relate to ownership of project and research outputs, compensation for community members time and efforts, hiring and retention practices of community members, equitable economic development initiatives, communication and for academic institutions appointment, promotion, and tenure requirements.

Democratization by institutions with communities attends to the equitable sharing of influence, power, and opportunity of institutional products such as knowledge, data, resources, and space. Institutes of higher learning hold an enormous abundance of knowledge, data, resources, and space of benefit to the community, community initiatives, and programs. To democratize is to open access to the community to the wealth of knowledge and expertise to redress social issues and generate life-changing technological and social innovation. The production and dissemination of knowledge is a power mechanism to unlock solutions that redress many of the disparities, inequities, and injustices communities face. Data animation and de-aggregation tells a fuller evidence-based truth of conditions and health of a community. It is democratized when translated into forms that are easily understood, readily available and accessible to stakeholders, decision-makers, and the community.

Along with policies come a variety of practices by institutional actors. Earlier, we discussed the role of the institutional actor in reifying institutional values through their behaviors. Therefore, it is important that practices are aligned with the ways of institutional being as they will be interpreted to reflect the values of the institution especially if demonstrated by many of its actors. Practices demonstrate to the community that what you mean in action is the same as what you say in words.

When engaging with communities, it is important to center the community expertise using that as the starting point to building out community engagement activities. If an institution is to do community engagement, then it is important to recognize community engagement as an act of partnership. You work with existing partners in various capacities which often might not center the institutions' needs but are toward the goal: to support, to listen, and to amplify. To be in partnership comes with expectation of democratization, reciprocity, and transparency. It also carries the responsibility of communicating and managing expectations.

Institutional practices that are counterproductive to healthy community engagement are those which are extractive and unsustained. Extractive practices are those where the institution takes what it needs from the community (knowledge, resources, innovation) without exchange, with inequitable exchange, and/or without mutual benefit. Seeking community knowledge, insight, and ideas are frequent conduct of academic institutions. With large education and research mandates, the academic enterprise relies on community participation and cooperation to help fulfill these central missions which make it vulnerable to falling into extractive patterns. Research and educational efforts produce programs, initiatives, new knowledge, and innovations that should benefit the communities who inspired and inform it. Furthermore, these outputs when introduced then not sustained—either started and stopped, funded and defunded, "feel" extractive, or impact trust. Therefore, partnership with other agencies and agency initiatives are critical to community engagement to ensure efforts are not siloed or duplicative and that capacity is built in to sustain efforts in collaboration.

6.5 Individual Ways of Being

For institutions to adopt these ways of being, the institutional actors must also adopt personal practices that are conducive to attaining good citizenship and healthy community engagement. Because structural racism is deeply embedded in all of our structures, individuals and healthcare providers, in particular, must be educated and practice as antiracists. Justice in Health calls out the racist practices that perniciously transcend healthcare practices and education to be uprooted. Implicit bias is frequently integrated into education and training of providers as a strategy to mitigate bias in providing care. Understanding how to be antiracist is a more forthright approach to combatting the issue of racism. It matches the energy of racism with the energy and tools to combat it. To be antiracist is to be "one who is supporting an antiracist policy through their actions or expressing an antiracist idea (Kendi, 2019, p. 13)." This antiracist idea is one that suggests any racial group as superior or inferior to another (Kendi, 2019, p. 20). Many resources (Wilkerson, 2020; Kendi, 2016, 2019) delve deeper into racism and its history which is beyond the scope of this chapter; however the responsibility for learning about it so as not to reify or adopt its practices is essential to being in communities especially those who are historically marginalized and underrepresented. Coming into the knowledge of history and how to function as an antiracist in society and in practice is what justice in health requires. Novak, Burnett and McCrea (2022) will release an interactive comprehensive antiracism education module for the education of healthcare professionals to promote diversity, equity, and belonging in healthcare education. Increasingly more and more professional associations offer antiracism position statements that are expected of their professionals, and this module will support the integration of these statements into action. Beyond the module is the need for curriculum transformation that is mirrored in licensure examination, institutional accreditation, and professional practice competencies. Otherwise these position statements are performative and lack the policy infrastructure and mandate for them to occur. While the approach thus far has been to recommend, changes in the profession will not happen organically across all of the interwoven stakeholders in professional education if not for a cohesive mandate and structure to ensure that it happens.

Individually, one can work to achieve a renewed awareness in their practice and seek out ways to include new approaches in their work and engagements with patients and the community. One of the practices that are important in this space is reflective practice of our being. Reflective practice allows for the intentional internal reflection and examination on our approaches, our behaviors, and our thoughts. To reflect is to peel back your way of being in interactions, in situations, your words, how you experienced moments/the day, and how you engaged across all of it. There is a bringing into awareness that reflection brings that must be actively sought; otherwise it is missed. Healthcare students are frequently assigned assignments where they write and submit reflective practice papers around an experience that evokes emotion, warrants introspection, or inquiry around its impact. We see students doing this when they have had a difficult clinical encounter and need to examine its effects on a personal level. It helps move toward an illuminated understanding of yourself and how to be better.

Tied closely to acts of reflection are mindfulness and appreciative inquiry both allow you to be present in moments with appreciation and valuing of its lessons. In mindfulness, you are intentionally present in your life, focused, and engaged so that you can bring the fullest of your functioning to bare in your interactions and engagements with undivided attentiveness. Appreciative inquiry speaks to demonstrating our valuing of others by asking questions that awakens appreciation to fuel truth seeking and innovative opportunities. Cooperrider and Fry (2020) state that it "involves, in a very artful and disciplined way, the craft of asking questions that elevate a system's cooperative capacity to apprehend strengths and positive potentials, unite around greater meanings and shared goals, and activate the kind of generative designs that serve to open those systems to better and more valued possibilities" (p. 267). There is a summoning of potential and a valuing of every resource within ourselves and each other that appreciative inquiry expects and that mindfulness and reflection helps us see.

6.5.1 Cultural Humility

Cultural humility is an important part of the diversity, equity, inclusion, and justice tapestry. Yet it is another term that is frequently used without clear consistent interpretation, prompting Foranda et al. (2016) to conduct a concept analysis of the term to clarify it. Their review of 62 articles on the topic reveal core attributes of cultural humility as openness, self-awareness, egoless, supportive interactions, self-reflection, and critique. Openness speaks to the receptivity to new ideas and diverse cultures. Self-awareness is the awareness of your own values, behaviors, and limitations. Egoless refers to humility and modesty while supportive interactions are positive exchanges and supportive engagements. Finally, self-reflection and critique is the act of reflecting on your thoughts and actions and together these attributes create a lifelong journey of transformative education, increased awareness, and humble exchanges (Foranda et al., 2016). From this holistic perspective, the understanding of cultural diversity is more expansive: it recognizes the unique experience of the individual as intersectional and context as a key influencer of those experiences (Fisher, 2020). According to Fisher (2020), "cultural humility focuses on developing characteristics that allow practitioners to approach individuals and situations with openness and awareness, to consider multiple perspectives simultaneously, and to use their positions to advocate for systemic change" (p. 57), Cultural humility inextricably connected to creating an inclusive culture. Generating a culture of inclusivity introduces difference and newness, allowing for diversity of thought, culture, experience, gender, and ethnicity. More and more organizations are operating with diversity, equity, and inclusion statements, missions, and entire offices. For organizations to achieve relative success in diversity, equity, and inclusivity efforts, its members and its actors need to be diverse and function inclusively and equitably.

Policies can only prescribe to a certain extent diversity measures, which are frequently narrowly relegated to the false construct of race and also by gender. Taken further, having more Black people and more women in an organization might create compositional diversity but how does it create inclusion? Are these individuals' equitable recipients of the organization's sense of belonging? Are they made to feel a welcome part of it by peers and leadership? To be inclusive, you must see yourself reflected in the institution and enjoy the celebration of your unique being. It's a practice that belongs to all members of the organization and is conveyed as a collective to the community with each encounter and interaction as a demonstration of how we value others.

6.6   Community Engagement as Ways of Doing

There are many ways of doing community-engaged work and there really is not a one-size-fits-all approach. Instead, there are practice principles for doing community-engaged work, irrespective of approach. At its simplest, community engagement cannot be viewed as an event. It is a process to be cultivated, nurtured, and sustained with the community at its center. This occurs through establishing bi-directional reciprocal relationships and partnerships with the community in all our engagement efforts.

Relationships and partnerships are the engines of community-engaged work. Relationships are built over time with the community and not emergent as a result of the institutional desires to have a community partner on a specific project. The most authentic relationships that can be built with communities are those that develop without intention of ever getting anything in return and those that are established over time. Relationships with community will require time and immersion in community spaces. To build and in most cases rebuild trust, the community needs to see trustworthy behaviors demonstrated consistently and over time which could take years. Keeping trust with the community is as important as building trust; hence many choices, actions, and decisions that seem to be harmless can destroy established relationships. Relationship building can also start by working in partnership with agencies and individuals who are already engaged with the community or populations in the community of interest. These agencies and individuals know who the community key stakeholders can give insight into approaches and community contacts essential to relationship building. Working in partnership with agencies also helps to align missions and efforts so that they are not duplicative in the community and overtaxing the same groups of individuals. This frequently happens when doing community-engaged research where several different schools and colleges may have various studies going on in a community while there are also students who are doing community practicums and other agencies and organizations implementing community programs. Without coordination and communication, these activities happen in siloes impacting the communities' perceptions of the institution and the communities' willingness to be involved now or in the future. Minimizing duplication of efforts and working in relation to and in partnership with the community and other agencies engaged with the community is an important step.

Another key act of partnership is that of sustainability. Initiatives, programs, and engagement with community must be planned for sustainability; otherwise a parachute in-and-out approach will be the default. While there are one-time events that might be required ultimately, they should be connected to a larger strategy that is sustained. Sustainability looks at inputs (resources, funding, and capacity), short-term and long-term, that allow for the activity/program/initiative to remain viable.

6.6.1   Community Leading the Way

Listening and responding to the needs of the community is a core nugget of community-engaged practice and research. The community is the expert and respecting them as such is demonstrated by the level of their inclusion from the beginning of the engagement process. Communities are acutely aware of their strengths and assets. They are the best source to identify opportunities, priorities, and offer ideas to address needs. When the foundation strategy FSG and Natrona Collective Health Trust (NCHT) recently partnered with the local community to devise a regional health equity plan, they stated:

"We also held focus groups with individuals who had lived experience: parents of small children, nonprofit leaders, youth, and advocacy and policy leaders. We prioritized listening to the voices we knew were most proximate to the issues. The community has the experience and up-close exposure to issues that external groups seek to understand and redress. Moreover, they can quickly identify potential missteps that institutional actors might make along the implementation pathway. Allowing community expertise to inform, direct, and influence is an investment in trust and fosters accountable practices" (Ridgway et al., 2021).

Community advisory boards have been established to help institutions navigate issues and approaches that are suitable to the community and supported by the community. A community advisor board is composed of community members with experience in the desired community who most often live, work, and serve in the community. These board members are brought together to guide and oversee a specific mission that the institution/agency or group is trying to implement in their community. Valuing the expertise of the community advisory board represents a willingness to connect and integrate the community voice first and foremost. Advisory board members should be compensated for their time because (1) they are providing a service that the institution is asking for and benefiting from and (2) those leading the project/initiative are getting paid for their time therefore it instills equity. Community advisory boards are not the only way to garner community input. Alternative structured approaches used to solicit community insight involve the use of focus groups, historical narratives, stories, interviews, and surveys. Focus groups and interviews are devised to systematically obtain information from the community through a planned platform that facilitates discussion. During either of these processes, the participants respond to guide questions about their perspectives and experiences to deepen understanding about opportunities and potential solutions. Surveys can also provide similar information and however are limited in their ability to explain the responses which are shaped by the survey design. The use of surveys with communities should be combined with another mechanism that elicits more in-depth information. Town hall meetings, stakeholder engagement sessions, and listening tours are loosely structured platforms that present opportunities for hearing from the community in an unfettered way.

Moving forward with any of these approaches comes with the responsibility of managing expectations with the community. Once you begin to solicit input from the community, it is already too late to try to manage expectations around what you intend to do with that input. Be clear and transparent upfront about the intention of obtaining the information, access to the information gathered, and how the information gathered will be used and shared back to the community. The institution should also be brought on board about expectations and agreement made before the information is gathered about all the aspects just identified. Communication with the community at all points of any engagement process helps hold space for transparency and trust. Keeping the community informed and involved in the way they would like to receive information is another important facet of doing community-engaged work. How institutions communicate and disseminate information does not always work for the community and nor does it happen where the community is.

Meeting the community where they are is not just a statement about the physical proximity to the community, it is also about the materials, the products, and the processes that are enacted in community engagement. Communication within the community makes use of what some institutions might view as non-traditional approaches such as in barbershops, churches, and at community events. However, these communal spaces are ideal for sharing important information, hosting programs, and connecting with the community.

Defining your community is to be considered when inviting community members to engage. Are you interested in a specific region, neighborhood, or population? Distill and be clear about who you are targeting. If it is a population, then know who the potential aggregate population within that group is that you are focused on. If it is a neighborhood, are there specific members of that neighborhood or boundaries that determine what constitutes the neighborhood? and then build out your strategies based on what you know and learn about that population. Be prepared and knowledgeable about your community before you engage with them. Learn the history, the stakeholders, previous efforts, findings, and outcomes from past initiatives, areas where of congregation? Insider versus outsider—which are you?

6.7 Social and Civic Innovation

Justice in health believes in the power of social and civic innovation to lead change. Community-engaged work generates civic innovation and social entrepreneurship—a brilliant by-product that leverages community-informed thought leadership in seeking impactful social solutions that are bold, new, and uniquely creative. It is a resetting of what is normative and courageously pursuing the unexplored or underexplored differently.

A recent story from Philadelphia showcased an organization called Fabric Health, a local start-up established to provide healthcare services to the community in laundromats (https://www.fastcompany.com/90717226/this-startup-is-turning-the-laundromat-into-the-doctors-office). Its co-founders identified the laundromat as a location where many lower-income families spend time weekly (upwards of 2 h per week) and partnered with local hospital and health insurance companies to offer health screening services onsite. They engage in "meeting families where they are in the time that they have" by greeting people and helping to carry laundry which then opens the door to health discussions (https://www.fabrichealth.org/). Important lessons from this exemplar demonstrate that community engagement can happen anywhere in the community creatively.

On a larger scale, Mastercard Center for Inclusive Growth (https://www.master-cardcenter.org/) provides equitable interventions pertaining to financial security, small business, and impact data. Their inclusive growth initiatives provide numerous examples of community engagement innovations that can yield results that benefit the community. One of their programs focus on partnership with other financial institutions to provide access to "Community Development Financial Institutions (CDFIs), including Community Reinvestment Fund USA (CRF) and Action Opportunity Fund, to integrate digital technologies and expand access to capital and programs for increasing numbers of women and entrepreneurs of color who have [been] disproportionately impacted by economic downturn brought on by COVID-19" (https://www.mastercardcenter.org/insights/helping-women-entrepreneurs-survive-and-thrive-in-the-digital-economy). The purpose of this community intervention is to overcome barriers to thriving among women entrepreneurs of color. These exemplars have shown us how to identify a community need that is addressed using community-based solutions that engage the members most affected by the issue and maximize impact. Less explored is the opportunity that technological innovation has to support the quest to ameliorate health inequity. Digital inequities are very present with access to basic technology such as the Internet and cellphones being problematic and unattainable to those with limited resources. Technological innovation can and should work in concert with social innovation to generate solutions. This will occur when knowledge is exchanged and co-created across transdisciplinary spaces and the space to do this has to be actively created and sought.

6.7.1 Being Strategic

Justice in health believes in community engagement as the way forward to address and mitigate health inequities and disparities. Even though community engagement is not new, the term is frequently used to convey any touchpoint with the community which creates misuse and misunderstanding of what community engagement really is. When operationalized optimally as outlined in this chapter, community engagement is the co-creation of community-centered solutions built upon community assets.

Many tools across various centers exist to help organizational preparedness and implementation of community engagement strategies. The World Health Organization provides global approaches to community engagement and a community engagement strategies checklist (https://apo.who.int/publications/i/item/9789240010529) for planning and thinking about your strategy. Texas A & M University offers community-engaged best practice recommendations with principles that can be readily adopted (https://ifsc.tamu.edu/Engagement) in the form of a community covenant. Their Institute for Sustainable Communities (IfSC) outlines parameters that address practices, processes, and reciprocal sharing for their covenant with the communities with which they engage.

Being strategic about your community engagement activities is to level set your intention with the needs of the community before jumping into community engagement work. Transparently provide as much information about the initiative, expectations, and deliverables at the onset. Leading up to that step you must first determine what is known and not known and how best to gather that information. Review historical documents, community demographic, and neighborhood level data from multiple sources to understand the determinants of health. Listen and learn from community stakeholders and begin to align your ideas with the information you are gathering. Integrate community members into the early stages of this process and work with them to identify the direction that is best for the community as determined by the community.

Conducting research with the community at inception becomes participatory and community engaged because it is co-created and implemented with the community. Being inclusive of your community involves sharing of power that weighs ideas, opinions, and resources equitably. Asking community members to participate should come with incentives that acknowledges their time and expertise as valuable and gives back to the individual and the community. This includes payment for time spent, using local business and hiring local labor as part of the initiatives, hosting in community spaces, leaving initiative materials and creations with the community. The democratized sharing of access, resources, and data with the community is another tangible opportunity to solidify your relationships with the community and demonstrate your values.

6.8   Communication and Dissemination Strategies

How information is shared with the community is critical to upholding the values of trust, transparency, and accountability. Communication with the community is a dialogue that is continuous and considerate of literacy, language, culture, and accessibility. When disseminating and sharing public health messages, it is important that the messaging is clear and at a literacy level which accommodates those at all levels of education. Be aware that there are recommended communication guidelines in some organizations that point to specific grade level targets for community facing communications which is fundamental to the exchange and translation of knowledge.

Many platforms for exchanging and translating knowledge exist, and some more than others are better suited for sharing information with the community. Each community is different and therefore their information sources also differ. Identifying the preferred way that your community is most likely to get information is the first consideration in any communication strategy. Churches, barbershops, community gathering spaces, neighborhood associations, key informants, and social media are communication avenues for information sharing. Every avenue requires a different process and messaging that fits with the platform. In some instances, communication can be in a flyer format; in other instances, it can be embedded in a QR code that is disseminated in high-touch community spaces. In person discussions at local sites, where individuals are verbally given information that they can then ask questions about, is also popular.

The use of creative platforms such as arts, plays, podcasts, and storytelling can engage the community in a more experiential way. Depending on your audience, opinion letters, policy briefs, and gray literature offer information and action around hot topics or current events. Each of these strategies are useful and most helpful when used in combination with each other and when targets for the appropriate audience. More formal knowledge dissemination strategies such as peer-reviewed journals, publications, and conference presentations are sought-after scholarly products in the research world but are not realistically useful for lay audiences.

Justice in health supports knowledge dissemination and translation in less hierarchical forms and welcomes a matrixed approach where a variety of platforms are used for outreach and knowledge exchange. Impact is not determined by journal rankings but by the scope and breadth of reach of the population for whom the work is intended to support. Policies that encumber the ability of scholars and practitioners to fully engage in community-engaged research and practice should be modified to accommodate for the uniqueness of this work.

6.9   Conclusion

Community-engaged work is not an event; it's a process and way of being. It creates an ecosystem of stakeholders galvanized by a similar sense of purpose and passion. Many of the points made focus on institutional community engagement efforts; however, the lessons identified here are transferable. The heartbeat of community-engaged work is centering the community as an equal partner in community solution-building. Being clear about what your intention for doing the work is before beginning this work is part of the preparation process for doing the work. Define and understand your community, its history, and its culture. Listen, include, and engage at the inception of your efforts and not once those efforts are already well underway or, worse, already completed. Many best practice approaches have been outlined that protect and support the community engagement process and avoid extractive, harmful behaviors. Those approaches start within the individual and are interdiscursively lined to the practices of the institution. There is no disconnect between the institution and its actors, only an extension of both that show up in practices, policies, and our values. Ongoing reflection by the institution and its constituents that allows for the necessary recalibrations along the way will help inadvertent missteps from reoccurring and preserve/restore trust. Keeping the trust of the community is as important as the effort to engage the community. The institution and its actors must be able to hold all engagement values while also doing the work with benevolence.

6.10   Reflective Questions and Considerations

1. What are some of the necessary pathways that need to be established in your work environment for you to authentically engage with the community? What is missing and how can it be implemented?
2. How does the practice of community engagement sustain the work that you do or how can it be used to enhance the work that is already being done?
3. Community engagement comes with many landmines and pitfalls? What are some of the ways in which they can be avoided and what should you do if they occur?
4. How can you use community-engaged approaches to impact change?
5. Write a draft charter that outlines how you and your organization demonstrate good citizenship with your community? Consider ways of being, knowing, and doing.
6. What does it mean to you to be a community solution-builder?

References

Bradberry, L. A., & De Maio, J. (2019). Learning by doing: The long-term impact of experiential learning programs on student success. *Journal of Political Science Education, 15*(1), 94–111.
Burnett, C., Swanberg, M., Hudson, A., & Schminkey, D. (2018, Winter). Structural justice: A critical feminist framework exploring the intersection between justice, equity and structural reconciliation. *Journal of Health Disparities Research and Practice, 11*(4), 52–68.
Cooperrider, D., & Fry, R. (2020). Appreciative inquiry in a pandemic: An improbable pairing. *The Journal of Applied Behavioral Science, 56*(3), 266–271. https://doi. org/10.1177/0021886320936265
Fabric Health. (2022). Retrieved May 2, 2022 from https://www.fabrichealth.org/
Fisher, E. S. (2020). Cultural humility as a form of social justice: Promising practices for global school psychology training. *School Psychology International, 41*(1), 53–66.
Foronda, C., Baptiste, D. L., Reinholdt, M. M., & Ousman, K. (2016). Cultural humility: A concept analysis. *Journal of Transcultural Nursing, 27*(3), 210–217.
Institute for Sustainable Communities. (2022a). *Engagement page*. Retrieved May 22, 2022, from https://ifsc.tamu.edu/Research-Ethics/Covenant-with-Communities

Institute for Sustainable Communities. (2022b) *Roles and responsibilities of the Institute of Sustainable Communities*. Retrieved May 22, 2022, from https://ifsc.tamu.edu/Research-Ethics/ Covenant-with-Communities

Kendi, I. (2016). *Stamped from the beginning*. Bold Type Books. ISBN 9781568584638.

Kendi, I. (2019). *How to be an antiracist.* . ISBN 9780525509295.

Lynch-Alexander, E. (2017). Defying the definition of insanity: Assessing the robust nature of University outreach in the community using carnegie Community engagement classification and Lynch Outreach Assessment Model (LOAM). *Journal of Academic Administration in Higher Education, 13*(1), 19–24.

Mastercard Center for Inclusive Growth. (2022a). Retrieved May 11, 2022, from https://www. mastercardcenter.org/

Mastercard Center for Inclusive Growth. (2022b). *Women's Empowerment: Helping women entrepreneurs survive and thrive in the digital economy*. Retrieved May 11, from https://www.mastercardcenter.org/insights/helping-women-entrepreneurs-survive-and-thrive-in-the-digital-economy

Mayne, Q., & Geibel, B. (2018, March). Don't good democracies need good citizens? Citizen dispositions and the study of democratic quality. *Politics and Governance, 6*(1), 33. https://doi. org/10.17645/pi1.1216

Novak, D., Burnett, C., & McCrea, L. (2022). *A New online module on antiracism and faculty, staff and trainee workshops to promote diversity, equity, and belonging in healthcare education*. Drexel University.

Peters, A. (2022). This start-up is turning the laundromat into the doctor's office. *Fast Company, Feb 2, 2022, World Changing Ideas*. Retrieved May 2, 2022, from https://www.fastcompany. com/90717226/this-startup-is-turning-the-laundromat-into-the-doctors-office

Ridgway, A., Kaika, A., & Cova, G. (2021). *How a new foundation utilized community voice in their strategy formation, 2021*. Retrieved May 19, 2022, from https://www.fsg.org/blog/ how-a-new-foundation-utilized-community-voice-in-their-strategy-formation/

Roberts, J. (2018). From the editor: The possibilities and limitations of experiential learning research in higher education. *The Journal of Experimental Education, 41*(1), 3–7.

Settles, I., Buchanan, N., & Dotson, K. (2019, August). Scrutinized but not recognized: (in)visibility and hypervisibility experiences of faculty of color. *Journal of Vocational Behavior, 113*, 62–74.

Settles, I., Jones, M., Buchanan, N., & Brassel, S. (2022). Epistemic exclusion of women faculty and faculty of color: Understanding scholar(ly) devaluation as a predictor of turnover intentions. *The Journal of Higher Education, 93*(1), 31–55. https://doi.org/10.1080/0022154 6.2021.1914494

Strum, S., Eatman, T., Saltmarch, J, & Bush, A. (2011) Full participation: Building the architecture for diversity and community engagement in higher education. *Imagining America, 17*. https:// surface.syr.edu/ia/17

The Association of Public and Land-grant Universities. (2022). *Commission on economic and community engagement*. Retrieved April 24, 2022, from https://www.aplu.org/ our-work/5-archived-projects/economic-development-and-community-engagement/

The Carnegie Foundation for the Advancement of Teaching. (2022). *Elective classification for community engagement document 2024 re-classification documentation guide to the application*. Retrieved April 24, 2022, from https://carnegieelectiveclassifications.org/wp-content/ uploads/2022/01/2024-Carnegie-Community-Engagement-Re-Classification-Guide.pdf

The Carnegie Foundation for the Advancement of Teaching Elective Classification. (2022). Retrieved April 24, 2022, from https://carnegieelectiveclassifications.org/ the-elective-classification-for-community-engagement-2/

Wilkerson, I. (2020). *Caste, the origins of our discontent*. Random House. ISBN 9780593230251.

World Health Organization. (2020). *Community engagement: A health promotion guide for universal health coverage in the hands of the people*. ISBN 978-92-4-001052-9 (electronic version). ISBN 978-92-4-001053-6 (print version). Retrieved May 2, 2022, from https://apo.who.int/ publications/i/item/9789240010529

Chapter 7
Just Health

This chapter summarizes and synthesizes the important points, complexities, and concepts raised throughout the previous chapters. It culminates in a discussion that pays particular attention to upstream versus downstream public and population health approaches to make the case as to why the reconciliation of public health toward just health cannot wait. Just health is revisited against this backdrop and summarized at the praxis of theory, knowledge, and action toward achieving health justice. The chapter concludes with a call to action and suggested steps to address the urgent and emergent conditions that mitigate health outcomes and identify opportunities for change that can be leveraged now.

7.1 The Recap

We started the *Justice in Health* journey with an overview and global introduction to the *Justice in Health* content by understanding core concepts of public health, equity, justice, and health that would be established. Early on, the focus was on unpacking the meaning of health, how health has been historically understood and misunderstood, and most importantly how health is created. This discussion offered a conceptual exploration of just health, and what the creation of a more just system of health means was introduced and situated in relation to our society and why health matters. Starting with understanding the common narrative has been a recurrent theme throughout the text emphasizing the importance of discourse and the role it plays in shaping how we conceive our practice and our solutions. Narratives and words are instrumental drivers of change and powerful conveyors of stories. Taking command of the narrative of health is a necessary part of any system change and crucial to making an impact. Getting to a common understanding around the

---

[1] Reprinted with permission from *Diverse: Issues In Higher Education*, www.DiverseEducation.com

language of health has to occur before we can set a common agenda for health and most importantly one that can truly improve lives and ameliorate disparities.

Chapter 2 took on the task of contextualizing and situating race and health in the United States. Knowing that the United States has increasing disparities and widening inequities along racialized lines introduced race as a factor warranting both examination and reflection. The history of subjugation, exclusion, and marginalization and its connection to much of the generational devastation to social, economic, and health outcomes was lifted up for awareness. There are much deeper discussions to be had, and many more historical exemplars than the ones discussed in Chap. 2 that support what is factually known: racialized populations disproportionately suffer from higher rates of several health-related (health disparities, chronic disease, morbidity, and mortality) and social consequences (such as poverty, limited access to opportunity, decrease social mobility, and racism) that diminish life expectancy and quality of life. Direct and indirect impacts of cumulative and intersecting exposure to these consequences produce chronic challenges that have been exacerbated by structures (institutions, policies, practices, and institutional agents), the inequitable distribution of power and privilege, and the history of race and health in this country. Healing in this country will only begin with truth and reconciliation, and this too must happen in the health professions and across all health disciplines. To get to truth, you must learn and engage in history and facts.

The Association of American Medical Colleges (AAMC) provides a resource list for those wanting to go deeper into the knowledge to explore race, power, and racism and recommended https://www.aamc.org/news-insights/racism-and-health-reading-list. Connecting the dots between the history and health disparities that are visible today is a necessary task for all health providers, decision-makers, and system actors. Harrell et al. (2011) article succinctly examines the multiple pathways that link racism to health outcomes offering models and processes that demonstrate social, psychological, and biological impacts and mediators.

In Chap. 3, we dove into frameworks for framing justice in health with a deeply philosophical introduction and exploration of key theories most critical to meet the health and well-being challenges we face as a nation. Highlighted were the discussions on critical theories and perspectives that included postcolonial and emancipatory inquiry, social justice in nursing practice, structural violence, and structural justice. Theory does more than philosophize ideas, it is a scaffolding for understanding and consolidating thoughts for application. Critical theory has been headlined with negative overtones. Justice in health takes an issue position that cannot be neutral in the midst of facts. The position on critical theory that embodies *Justice in Health* is that critical inquiry encourages criticism, interrogation, and deconstruction necessary to actualize justice and humanity for all. It is believed that both justice and humanity are inalienable rights that are bestowed to all irrespective of status, ethnicity, identity, and location. Accountability ensures that this happens, and critical inquiry is the instigative approach to determining if it has happened and urges action to make it happen. Discussion about the social determinants of health was explored to help bring into awareness the contextual causes that determine health guided by these various theoretical perspectives. In doing so, Justice in

Health served to synthesize structural and root causes through exposing the hidden realities of power, privilege, and social identity.

With those chapters laying foundation information needed to engage with confidence in cogent discourse on equity, Chap. 4 spotlights critical health equity and issues by exposing critical root causes that perpetuate health disparities such as racism, poverty, mass and youth incarceration, violence against women, communities, and society. Select equity issues that determine health such as access to care, access to opportunity, and other determinants where profiled using concrete examples. Beyond identification of these issues, the practical examples served to make the connection to the earlier perspectives more visible and further extend and situate health in relation to structural drivers and root causes. The act of connecting the dots outside of the current orientation of health leads to a deeper understanding of how health happens across disparate populations and within aggregate populations. It should also begin to stand up the framing for what an equitable systems approach could look like and what must be considered.

By Chap. 5, the notion of creating a healthcare system without walls to build a culture of healing was proposed. It intentionally starts to shift current held beliefs of what a healthcare system is, toward what it could be conceptualized as the building of a system of care without walls. To build a healthcare system without walls, current structural obstacles, and gaps including their impacts and while introducing new ways to overcome and dismantle these challenges is recommended. Critical conversations have to entail what it means to be a healthcare provider and how we can better prepare healthcare providers to meet the demands of a new reimagined system. This includes introducing trauma-informed approaches, which are highlighted as one of many key professional shifts required in the routine preparation of healthcare providers. Trauma impacts individuals and community which makes use of trauma-informed approaches in support of healing an essential part of any strategy. It is a required overarching mechanism for facilitating and creating a culture of healing in and beyond our systems of care.

Community engagement and partnerships are explored in Chap. 6 to achieve just action to facilitate the rebuilding and co-creating a system of care. Understanding community partnership and their importance has been discussed and best practice principles for engaging with the community to meet their health needs where they are emphasized. Exemplars from the field that demonstrate authentic community engagement and partnership exemplars taught us how communities can mobilize and transform health. Chapter 6 served to help health providers, health researchers, and health educators consider non-traditional approaches to creatively find ways to exchange knowledge, skills, and expertise needed to reform and redress health disparities. It is a chapter to encourage healthcare providers to act effectively in partnership to create and influence equitable health solutions.

The book concludes with this chapter—Chap. 7 on "Just Health"—that serves to summarize and synthesize the important points, complexities, and concepts raised throughout the previous chapters. It culminates in a discussion that pays particular attention to upstream versus downstream public and population health approaches to make the case as to why the reconciliation of public health toward just health cannot wait.

7.2   Context Driving Care

Justice in Health believes in health that is just and sovereign. It has redefined health to encompass multiple ways of knowing what health is and various ways of doing that work in tandem toward a shared common goal of intentionally creating health equity. Health equity is not homogenous in its application across all groups because disparities vary within and between populations based on many of the factors examined throughout this text. Justice-in-health approaches accelerate solutions prioritized to suit populations that need it most and addresses them in partnership with and informed by the population of focus. Since a justice-in-health approach values the community expertise and the community's traditions, the bar determining what is equitable and just health is co-created with the community. Outcomes that reflect health sovereignty in experiences, access to opportunity and innovation, and access to care and resources and that improve the quality and outcomes of life at the root are expected with this lens. Establishing the bold vision of justice in health must allow and generate autonomy where fluidity of experiences, varying interpretations of thriving, and intersecting health identities co-exist amidst equitable structures.

Above all else, the pursuit of health justice is the achievement of health sovereignty which without compromise recognizes the inherent right of health and that of humanity to converge and then support its ability to flourish. This book has emphasized: (a) interrogating and deconstructing health narratives; (b) the inextricable link between history, context, and the individual; and (c) the pursuit of structural reimagination and transformation of health care in the United States. Just health is an ontological call to action driven by the urgency of now which has presented itself as multiple pandemics: COVID-19, persistent racial injustice, and perpetual and increasing health disparities, each standing as intersecting issues in relation to each other. Multidimensional actions are required and a plan that considers how and where those actions need to occur must begin. Justice in health suggests critical high touchpoints where action plans can focus which include the radical re-education of our healthcare providers and rapid structural reform of the current healthcare system.

Tangential to these points are the state of our system of care and the stark reality of its ineffectiveness to mitigate health inequity and disparity and failure to provide accessible care to all. COVID-19 seemed to be the tipping point that caused more attention to be given to the state of the healthcare system because of the burden it placed on its operations and ability to function. More proactive motivation to change the system must happen and that motivation has to be primarily driven with an eliminating health disparities vision versus continuing to treat the disparities. That reactive approach feels irrational and given the rising healthcare costs, widening health disparities, and increasing chronic diseases, they simply are not sustainable. While there are other system layers at issue which also need to be addressed such as its complex reimbursement and administration structures, its dominant tertiary focus, and the influence of key stakeholders, what still holds true is that it needs to change. We need to stop talking about change, researching change, and make the change that we already know needs to be made.

The reckoning of the pandemics in this nation has awoken an urgency to act; and as with other significant moments in history, that window will close. Before it does, there is no reason why healthcare system actors, providers, and stakeholders cannot be mobilized to act, to reimagine, and to restructure. This book intentionally started the conversation of health focused on defining health by examining historical policy statements that were ratified by the United States as acts of agreement. We must hold our system accountable to functioning from a place that honors those commitments and view of what health is and use that as the platform to imagine what it should be.

Justice in Health proposes a radical vision for health in the absence of one being articulated that attempts to address the habitual inequities borne primarily at the expense of disparate populations. Continuing to accept the current system as one that can structurally optimize health equitability is to be complicit. As healthcare providers, we must engineer a system that works for all. This can be done. Our values are reflected in our actions and inaction. Justice in health stands on the side of action and seeks to eliminate excuses by illuminating possibility through daring to examine innovative solutions.

We have seen the aspirational messages and the call to actions by institutions, professional organizations, and even our government—many of which have been included in the preceding chapters. However, dialogue *about* action must be combined *with* action as necessary ingredients for change. What has not been discovered is an action plan and road map to dismantle and restructure the system, not to mention any allocated budget to make this happen. While daunting, it is possible. In the height of frustration during the pandemic, I wrote an Op-Ed "The Afterthought of Equity" in attempting to speak truth to power and ignite conversations that offer concrete structural actions (see Box 7.1 for full text). As an act of critical caring, I had borne witness to too much to be silent and still carry the weight of that responsibility to find a way to galvanize and activate some sort of meaningful change. Justice in health is one way and I am sure there are others.

Because healthcare providers are bearing witness to injustice in health and are on the frontlines of treating many health disparities, we must be involved in policy and advocacy now more than ever. Health is political and many health inequities are codified through legislation, regulations, and appropriations. COVID-19 vaccine distribution; abortion rights; the Special Supplemental Nutrition Program for Women, Infants, and Children (WIC) (US Government USDA, 2022b); US Department of Housing and Urban Development (HUD) (US Government HUD, 2022a); Violence Against Women's Act (US Government White House, 2022a); and recently the Inflation Reduction Act (US Government White House, 2022b) are all examples of health policies that have the power to eliminate or perpetuate disparity. Engaging in the political arena is not for everyone and that is not what is being proposed. What should be expected of every provider is basic knowledge and skills of advocacy and an awareness of health policy (in their organizations, communities, and/or at various levels of government) and its role in relation to health issues and health equity.

At a minimum, knowledge and awareness of these and other pertinent health policies and its impacts should be the standard for those who work within and in collaboration with health care. With the extent of disparities known and established, particularly in health, ask who has taken leadership and responsibility for doing an equity analysis of policies that perpetuate health disparities and examine the intended and unintended consequences of their implementation? Is there a professional body, consortium, or an office, governmental or otherwise, that has taken on this important charge as a core part of its mandate? There should be, and if not, this should be of deep concern to all health providers because of the far-reaching impact that health inequity and disparities have on the practice of health care, the delivery of care, and in the lives of the community. The outcry should be so strong making it unavoidable to ignore, yet it is not. Meanwhile, rates of preventable diseases are exceedingly high and life expectancy exceedingly low for the most vulnerable populations and have been proven to be solely based along lines of race and census tract. We know what the issues are, for whom, and where they are most prolific. Sit with that for a moment. It is incognizable. Where is the righteous indignation?

Heather Heyer gave her life standing up to racial injustice in Charlottesville, Virginia, in 2017, when White supremacists from across the United States converged on the quaint southern city for a rally (https://www.bbc.com/news/world-us-canada-40924922). Heather's last Facebook post said—*if you are not outraged, you're not paying attention* (https://www.bbc.com/news/world-us-canada-40924922). We need to be outraged to act and galvanize our efforts and attention toward collective action with a common goal of creating a healthcare system that is equitable and just.

Box 7.1: The Afterthought of Equity (Op-Ed) (Burnett, 2021)[1]

Dismantling racism is going to take far more than branding the word, "equity". Equity demands work that will not be solved by simply adding the word to your strategic plan or initiatives so you can check mark it off your lists. So, let's take an honest look at how we can really begin to do this work, in earnest.

Calls for equity culminated amidst the backdrop of last summer's horrific on and off camera killings of Black people overlaid by COVID's illumination of widening disparities. This has rightly amplified cries for not just equity but for justice. Yet there is a discomforting disingenuity that I feel as a Black woman, a nurse scientist and scholar, when repeatedly the responses to predictable inequity occur after the fact. Instead, they are reactive attempts at equity that are fundamentally flawed. Using the now widely and wildly popular 'equity brand' is counter-intuitive to acting on equity simply by its passive implementation.

It is obvious to those of us who live, breath and experience inequity daily, that equity remains an afterthought. A primary example of this is a January 2021 Kaiser Health News report citing lower COVID-19 vaccination rates for Black, Indigenous, Latinx, and People of Color than Whites—by as much as 50 percent or more in some regions. Further, a recent U.S. National Academy of Sciences report estimated that COVID-19 induced reductions in the life expectancy of Black and Latino populations are three to four times less than that of Whites—a trend which is expected to persist and undo the last 10 years of progress (Andrasfay & Goldman, 2021). Both issues are seeded in the structural manifestations of racism, inequity, and injustice. What's worse is

(continued)

Box 7.1 (continued)

that these gaps in existing and new inequities within these specific popula-tions have been scientifically documented and well known for decades.

Therefore, inequity when left unaddressed, will continue to surface, and resurface. So while we purport to care about equity, and are deeply incensed by the unjust consequences of its absence, we still refuse to co-create struc-tures, systems and policies where equity is embedded from the beginning and not tacked on after. We cannot retrofit equity into inequitable structures.

This is not a criticism of the well-intended and much needed equity efforts; it is a critique of the ineptitude of the broader structural processes to mitigate and ameliorate equity and create justice.

Focusing on structures as the starting point for solutions is key because much of these disparities and inequities are deeply embedded in root causes housed within and often perpetuated by structures, their systems, policies and practices. Most importantly, there is a predictability in the anticipation of inequity that should force us to proactively prepare to address it before it manifests instead of waiting until it does. Otherwise, we will once again begin the same cycle of trying to scramble to equalize the issue and create equity in the moment and worst after the inequity has already occurred.

What must happen is moving equity as an afterthought to equity as the default, so that it's a proactive solution instead of a reactive one. Doing 'some-thing' does not mean we are doing all that we can do. Inequity must be treated with urgency and intensity like the existential threat that is it.

Beyond using an 'equity lens' in a siloed patchwork approach, we must co-create and animate equity everywhere. Our structures have to be re-mantled toward structural justice (Burnett et al., 2018). Structural spaces are where inequity, injustice and racism have been insidiously internalized. It is where community trust has been historically broken and detrimentally harmed in communities of color.

Therefore, we need designated equity centers, offices, and departments of equity, created nationwide led by equity and community experts, to examine and lead these efforts up close. Mobilizing true equity is a long-haul, broad sweeping strategic effort. It's not a report, a committee, nor a taskforce. Funded leadership and offices at the state, local and national level with an endorsed equity mandate that is empowered to coordinate efforts to actively address and cultivate equity across all our sectors, systems, policies, and pro-cedures is desperately needed.

Without this radically reimagined approach to redressing inequity, equity will remain elusive as a patchwork brand symbolically pulled out as needed with no real process or concerted strategy. Equity will continue as an after-thought until we intentionally incubate, embed, and implement innovative equitable solutions at multiple levels.

Redressing inequity once it occurs is still important, however so too is preventing inequity from occurring in the first place. Both are necessary acts of justice making. The work is just starting.

7.3   Solutions: *Justice in Health* Action Plan

To imagine a plan for action, steps to ignite and lead reform starts with affirming the intellectual (i.e., includes high professional standards, rigorous academic scholarship; making space for clients to engage in their own problem-solving and critical thinking; engages multicultural perspectives; etc.) and the spiritual (i.e., honors our humanity; instills a sense of wonder, sacredness, and humility in our practice settings; respects and embraces alternate cultural realities; the involvement of social change and healing; and the interconnectedness of practitioners and clients in meaningful ways), with a firmly entrenched culture of the academy that supports our professional practice as well as our personal practices. It also involves the concrete—the co-creating equitable and just structures and necessary steps and strategies for making that happen. "The Afterthought of Equity" is an attempt to inspire and ignite reform and its sentiment has evolved into the grounding of a Justice-in-Health discourse about how to catalyze momentum. Considering all of the elements that operationalize the healthcare machine is beyond the scope of the vision of these catalyzing solutions. However, those select solutions which are offered here are focused on major system facilitators that must be engaged in shaping a new way forward.

7.3.1   Structural Reimagination

If nothing else, it is hoped that *Justice in Health* sounded another alarm about the urgent need for structure change, now. Proposed are some high-level considerations to help facilitate this change and that focus on unified approaches to the patchwork and siloed nature of the work, of philosophies, and of missions.

- Truth and Reconciliation Commission in the United States should be established. The history of racial injustice is lengthy and rooted in everything that we experience now and in the future. Denial of its impact is not a solution, acknowledgment toward healing is. Truth and Reconciliation Commissions have been established in countries that also have a history of racial injustice such as Rwanda (https://www.nurc.gov.rw/index.php?id=69) and Canada (https://nctr.ca/about/history-of-the-trc/truth-and-reconciliation-commission-of-canada/) to raise awareness and promote healing and unity through many initiatives.
- A National Health Equity and Justice Commission and a common new agenda for health and health equity has to be set for the United States with a clear mission, mandate for the re-envisioning of health in the United States, and setting of a community agenda for health and health equity. It would serve as a centralized collaborating center for health equity with an Office that houses the preceding items (National Health Equity Plan, Health Equity Technical and Expert Support, and Database and Evaluation of National Health Equity Best Practices, National office for subsequent regional and state health equity offices.

- National Health Equity Plan: The creation of a multicomponent national plan that includes an implementation plan (with resource allocation and assigned leadership and targeted best practice strategies with outcome impacts and targets and robust communication strategy). The plan needs to embed an evaluation strategy and include necessary steps of asset assessment (what programs and initiatives are already working well that can be scaled and embedded into strategies), structural assessment (policies, procedures, and practices with recommendations and mechanisms for change), timelines, and accountability (including impact measures). Health equity and health justice in all policies is suggested as core principles for the strategy as are offices and designation of health equity actors in each state that oversee the implementation and evaluation of the strategy. Connection and collaboration with key health equity research and strategy organizations (Robert Wood Johnson Foundation (RWJF), Aspen Institute, National Institutes of Health (NIH), Ford Foundation, Professional Health Associations, Quality Improvement and For/Non-profit organizations (such as racial justice and health equity organizations) and others have to occur, orchestrated through the commission or an assigned entity. Building an equity consortium/network of partners by establishing a community of scholars, community members, organizations, and practitioners who can cross-pollinate ideas and innovation, share transdisciplinary expertise, and offer supportive guidance is needed.
- National and Community Advisory Groups to offer guidance and expert advice to the Commission and regional offices and most importantly invite the recipients of care into the conversation and engage the communities that we are serving. Having buy-in and expert community guidance is critical to reform and change of any service or system.

We have to recalibrate the current system led by public and population health objectives, impact measures, and expected outcomes across all health settings.

7.3.2 Healthcare Providers

All providers need to seize the moment and opportunity to lead and repurpose our practice mission as clinicians, scientists, and educators. In today's climate, Americans have an extraordinary amount of distrust in our systems and institutions. And for 19 years and counting, nursing remains the nation's most-trusted profession. It only makes sense that we tap into this trust and recognize more nurses as leaders and decision-makers in our healthcare, education, and government systems.

By elevating our nurses, we elevate all other health providers and elevate the health of our nation. Nurses have a diverse skill set (scientists, practitioners, health advocates, community engagers), practice in settings ranging from hospital to homes, and are educated with a holistic orientation of health (social determinants of health, drivers of health, biological, physiological, and mental health), not to mention have the founding principle of social justice as their practice. Therefore, it is proposed that centering of nurse's historical legacy and expertise be used to help lead health system reform and transform our systems of care by recommending:

- The elevation of a chief nursing officer position and an equity engagement officer across each state and territories to work in collaboration with health centers, hospitals, institutions, public health departments, and communities.
- The infusion of nursing equity expertise and community engagement to inform plans and policies that encompass issues of social justice, equity, and health challenges facing our society today.
- A much wider representation of all disciplines, on all existing government and regional task forces and commissions to provide an equity lens and a critical look at where opportunities exist for structural reform and measures to mitigate disparities.
- The integration of better practice approaches of:
- Health Screening and Intervening for the social determinants of health as a practice standard by all.
- Health equity into all policies and practices.
- Trauma-informed care and healing approaches across the system.
- Centering the community as experts to humanize care and care interactions.
- Transdisciplinary education, research, training and innovation.

7.3.3   Provider Education

Preparing the next generation of healthcare providers with an orientation of social justice, founded on the unwavering belief that health is a right is one of the most important acts of justice making we can do. We have not and will continue not to make progress in the eradication of health disparities and inequities until the collective "we" get on the same page about the basics of health, including its definition and it as a right. Any profession that has the privilege of engaging with individuals seeking health have to educate with consensus around this very basic yet fundamental principle.

- Curriculum Transformation: Aim for transformative curriculum development by enacting key initiatives and education in community engagement, history of community, history of medical and mistrust, racism and antiracism in health, and ending the use and teaching of race-based clinical decision models (including calculators).
- Antiracism: It has been empirically proven and substantiated that health disparities occur along lines of marginalization particularly those of race and ethnicity. This has not changed for decades and in fact they have worsened. Those in practice should receive antiracist education and training routinely from pre-licensure through including post-licensure. This along with diversity, equity, and inclusion must become an established measurable practice competency required of all accredited healthcare schools and licensure examination that is expected and evaluated.

- Entry to Practice Licensure Examination: For healthcare professionals, there is the need to put weight of equal importance and significance on the social determinants of health, diversity, equity, and inclusion as there is on the physical health aspects of identification and treatment of disease.
- Accreditation bodies that oversee health professional training and education programs should set evaluation standards that include multi-year curriculum audits that demonstrate evidence of training and practice experience in the social determinants of health, diversity, equity and inclusion, and in trauma-informed and antiracist approaches. This training should be evident throughout all curriculum threads.
- Transdisciplinary Training and Research are practice essentials needed to structurally address the ongoing challenges of inequity and disparity and to practice within a *Justice-in-Health* framework. Overcoming barriers to transdisciplinary research, community-engaged research, and transdisciplinary practice must be identified and solutions to overcome them implemented. Social and technological innovation to ameliorate inequities has to be at the forefront of training and research activities that must occur within transdisciplinary community-engaged teams. The issues are not siloed, and therefore neither can our professional preparation and practice.
- Recruitment and Retention of underrepresented faculty, students, and providers are an important priority and instrumental to any strategy to address health disparities and promote equity. Identification and implementation of strategies that support both retention and recruitment of underrepresented faculty, students, and providers have to be applied across settings. Obstacles to access opportunities for enrollment, professional advancement, and leadership should be removed. More diverse representation in leadership in health institutions, government appointments, research, and organizations is an important catalyst for sustained change.

7.4 Conclusion and Reaffirmation

As healthcare professionals, we must build and lead across disciplines and coalitions to reshape and transform health care toward more equitable and just spaces. We are in desperate need of the launch of a National Healthcare System Re-Imagination Strategy and a critically conscious group of healthcare providers and community members to move boldly into accelerated action. While there are massive logistical considerations for how to make this happen, the initiation of thinking about making this happen should occur. Presently we have a Cancer Moonshot to rid our nation of the scourge of cancer once and for all; however, this can never be a reality when cancer disparities exist and persist. Until we address health disparities and create health justice, no amount of moonshot initiatives, regardless of how well intended, will ever work. If we can run a successful space race, allocate billions of dollars toward chronic diseases, we can exert the same fervent energy to ameliorate health disparities. Chapter 4 raised the proposition of a national health dialogue and action plan. This must unequivocally happen and orbit around the health as humanity strategy where we implement a process for both dialogue and strategy clearly outlining expectations and outcomes; define what health is and be clear about where health happens; fearlessly explore all opportunities for health and health services across locations/settings; seek to reimagine our existing system toward a system integrated with population and public health; embed health and equity in all of our policies; and entrench accountable stewardship for health in structural oversight bodies and offices of health equity and justice in every department. Creating *Justice in Health* is a national emergency to which a far-reaching response is warranted at a scale that echoes the situation and our expressed desires to change it. It is simply insufficient to stay in a perpetual state of mitigating harm; you must do good and work to prevent it in the process.

References

American Association of Medical Colleges. Retrieved July 1, 2022 from: https://www.aamc.org/news-insights/racism-and-health-reading-list).

Andrasfay, T., & Goldman, N. (2021). Association of the COVID-19 pandemic with estimated life expectancy by race/ethnicity in the United States, 2020. *JAMA Network Open, 4*(6), e2114520. https://doi.org/10.1001/jamanetworkopen.2021.14520

BBC News. (2017). *Who is Heather Heyer?* Retrieved May 20, 2022, from https://www.bbc.com/news/world-us-canada-40924922

Burnett, C. (2021, March 4). *The afterthought of equity. Diverse: issues in higher education.* Retrieved May 12, 2022, from https://www.diverseeducation.com/covid-19/article/15108719/the-afterthought-of-equity

Burnett, C., Swanberg, M., Hudson, A., & Schminkey, D. (2018, Winter). Structural justice: A critical feminist framework exploring the intersection between justice, equity and structural reconciliation. *Journal of Health Disparities Research and Practice, 11*(4), 52–68.

Government of Canada. (2022). *National Commission on truth and reconciliation of Canada.* Retrieved July 4, 2022, from https://nctr.ca/about/history-of-the-trc/truth-and-reconciliation-commission-of-canada/

Harrell, C. J., Burford, T. I., Cage, B. N., Nelson, T. M., Shearon, S., Thompson, A., & Green, S. (2011, April 15). Multiple pathways linking racism to health outcomes. *Du Bois Review, 8*(1), 143–157. https://doi.org/10.1017/S1742058X11000178. PMID: 22518195. PMCID: PMC3328094.

Republic of Rwanda. (2022). *National Unity and Reconciliation Commission.* Retrieved July 4, 2022, from https://www.nurc.gov.rw/index.php?id=69

United States Government. (2022a). *US Department of Housing and Urban Development.* Retrieved from: https://www.hud.gov/

United States Government. (2022b). *The special supplemental nutrition program for Women, Infants, and Children (WIC).* Retrieved July 4, 2022, from https://www.fns.usda.gov/wic

Whitehouse Government. (2022a). *Reauthorization of the violence against women's' act.* Retrieved July 4, 2022, from https://www.whitehouse.gov/briefing-room/statements-releases/2022/03/16/fact-sheet-reauthorization-of-the-violence-against-women-act-vawa/

Whitehouse Government. (2022b). *State fact sheets: How the inflation reduction act lowers health care costs across America.* Retrieved August 22, 2022, from whitehouse.gov/briefing-room/statements-releases/2022/08/18/state-fact-sheets-how-the-reduction-act-lowers-health-care-costs-across-america/.

Appendix: Resource List by Topic

Health Equity

CDC: Health equity resources (information and strategies)

https://www.cdc.gov/nccdphp/dnpao/health-equity/health-equity-resources.html

CDC: Tools for putting Social Determinants of Health (SDOH) into action (resource for practitioners to take action)

https://www.cdc.gov/socialdeterminants/tools/index.htm

CDC: Youth Health and Educational Disparities (action steps, considerations and resources)

https://www.cdc.gov/healthyyouth/disparities/action.htm

American Public Health Association: Creating the Healthiest Nation – Opportunity Youth

https://www.apha.org/-/media/Files/PDF/topics/equity/Opportunity_Youth.ashx

American Public Health Association: Health Equity Resources

https://www.apha.org/topics-and-issues/health-equity

The Commonwealth Fund: Health Equity Featured Stories

https://www.commonwealthfund.org/health-equity

Kaiser Family Foundation: Data dashboards, information and highlights on health policy and racial equity

https://www.kff.org/racial-equity-and-health-policy/

U.S. Department of Health and Human Services, National Institute on Minority Health and Health Disparities: The PhenX social determinants of health assessments collection

C. Burnett, *Justice in Health*, https://doi.org/10.1007/978-3-031-18504-5

https://www.nimhd.nih.gov/programs/collab/phenx/index.html

U.S. Department of Health and Human Services, Office of Disease Prevention and Health Promotion: Healthy People 2030 National Objectives for Health

https://health.gov/healthypeople

U.S. Department of Health and Human Services, Office of Disease Prevention and Health Promotion: Healthy People 2030 National Objectives for Health Equity

https://health.gov/healthypeople/priority-areas/health-equity-healthy-people-2030

WHO: Health Equity Assessment Toolkit (assessment of health equity tools)

https://www.who.int/data/inequality-monitor/assessment_toolkit

WHO: Health Inequality Monitor – Health Equity Visualization (interactive data visualization platform)

https://www.who.int/data/inequality-monitor

Racial Equity

American Public Health Association: Advancing Racial Equity Webinar Series

https://www.apha.org/Events-and-Meetings/Webinars/Racial-Equity

American Public Health Association: Racism and Health Webinar Series

https://www.apha.org/Events-and-Meetings/Webinars/Racism-and-Health

American Public Health Association: *Racism: Science and Tools for the Public Health* Professional (Book)

https://secure.apha.org/imis/ItemDetail?iProductCode=978-087553-3032 &CATEGORY=BK

Building Healthy Places Network: Healthy Neighborhood Investments Policy Scan and Strategy Map – Community-led policy-setting tool to address inequity

https://www.buildhealthyplaces.org/tools-resources/healthy-neighborhood-investments-policy-scan/

CDC: Racial and Ethnic Approaches to Community Health (REACH)

https://www.cdc.gov/nccdphp/dnpao/state-local-programs/reach/

The Color of Care (Documentary)

https://www.thecolorofcare.org/

The Commonwealth Fund: Racial and Ethnic Equity Scorecard

https://www.commonwealthfund.org/publications/scorecard/2021/nov/achieving-racial-ethnic-equity-us-health-care-state-performance

Prevention Institute: Building Bridges: The Strategic Imperative for Advancing Health Equity and Racial Justice

https://www.preventioninstitute.org/publications/building-bridges-strategic-imperative-advancing-health-equity-and-racial-justice

Community Engagement
U.S. Department of Health and Human Services, National Institutes of Health: Principles of community engagement, 2nd Edition

https://www.atsdr.cdc.gov/communityengagement/pdf/PCE_Report_508_FINAL.pdf

Moving Health Care Upstream: The Engine of Population Health Networks: Understanding & Using Integrative Activities – Integrator Learning Lab

https://www.movinghealthcareupstream.org/collection/

Moving Health Care Upstream: Population Health Integrators

https://www.movinghealthcareupstream.org/population-health-integrators/

Patient-Centered Outcomes Research Institute (PCORI): Engagement Resources https://www.pcori.org/engagement/engagement-resources
Neighborhood Resilience Project

https://neighborhoodresilience.org/

Health Profession Resources
American Nurses Association: Elevate your awareness of racism in nursing: Resources for change

https://www.nursingworld.org/practice-policy/workforce/clinical-practice-material/national-commission-to-address-racism-in-nursing/resources-for-change/

American Medical Association: Health Equity CME and Education Resources

https://www.ama-assn.org/delivering-care/health-equity/health-equity-cme-education-resources

American Medical Association: The AMA's Organizational Strategic Plan to Embed Racial Justice and Advance Health Equity 2021–2023

https://www.ama-assn.org/about/leadership/ama-s-strategic-plan-embed-racial-justice-and-advance-health-equity

American Nurses Association: Foundational Report on Racism in Nursing

https://www.nursingworld.org/practice-policy/workforce/clinical-practice-material/national-commission-to-address-racism-in-nursing/commissions-foundational-report-on-racism%2D%2Din-nursing/

The Commonwealth Fund: Confronting Racism in Health Care

https://www.commonwealthfund.org/publications/2021/oct/confronting-racism-health-care

National Academies of Sciences, Engineering, and Medicine: The Future of Nursing 2020–2030: Charting a Path to Achieve Health Equity

https://www.nationalacademies.org/event/05-11-2021/the-future-of-nursing-2020-2030-charting-a-path-to-achieve-health-equity-report-release-webinar

World Innovation Summit for Health: Nurses for Health Equity: Guidelines for Tackling the Social Determinants of Health (PDF)

https://www.wish.org.qa/reports/nurses-for-health-equity-guidelines-for-tackling-the-social-determinants-of-health/

References

Government of the United States Department of Health and Human Services. (2022a). *Healthy people 2030*. Retrieved July 9, 2022, from https://health.gov/healthypeople

Government of the United States Department of Health and Human Services. (2022b). *Health equity in healthy people 2030*. Retrieved July 9, 2022, from https://health.gov/healthypeople/priority-areas/health-equity-healthy-people-2030

United Nations. (2022a). *Department of Economic and Social Affairs. Sustainable development goal one*. Retrieved July 8, 2022, from https://sdgs.un.org/goals/goal1

United Nations. (2022b). *Department of Economic and Social Affairs. Sustainable development goal two*. Retrieved July 8, 2022, from https://sdgs.un.org/goals/goal2

Index

© The Editor(s) (if applicable) and The Author(s), under exclusive license to
Springer Nature Switzerland AG 2022
C. Burnett, *Justice in Health*, https://doi.org/10.1007/978-3-031-18504-5

Printed in the United States
by Baker & Taylor Publisher Services